D0302483

# Understanding
# Cholesterol

Dr Mike Laker

Published by Family Doctor Publications Limited
in association with the British Medical Association

© Family Doctor Publications 2000–2008
Updated 2003, 2006, 2008

Family Doctor Publications, PO Box 4664, Poole, Dorset BH15 1NN

ISBN-13: 978 1 903474 17 4
ISBN-10: 1 903474 17 5

# Contents

# About the author

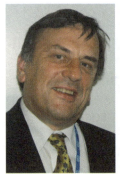

**Dr Mike Laker** is Medical Adviser to the North East Strategic Health Authority and Honorary Reader in Clinical Biochemistry at the University of Newcastle upon Tyne. He has extensive experience in cholesterol and fat metabolism, with particular interests in their relationship to coronary heart disease and diabetes mellitus. He is a past Secretary of the British Hyperlipidaemia Association.

# Introduction

## What is cholesterol and why does it matter?

Cholesterol is a type of fat (lipid) that is found in your blood and every cell of your body. It is important because high levels of cholesterol in your blood increase your risk of developing coronary heart disease (CHD) – one of the most common causes of death and disability in Europe, North America and Australia.

## How common is coronary heart disease?

In the UK, about 26 per cent of deaths in men and 19 per cent of deaths in women under the age of 75 years are now caused by CHD, with another 13 to 14 per cent resulting from other related conditions affecting the heart and blood vessels.

## What is the pattern of coronary heart disease?

High rates of CHD occur particularly in the developed world, where lifestyle and dietary factors play important contributory roles. Within Europe, the incidence of CHD is higher in northern than in Mediterranean countries, and this difference is thought to be the result of dietary factors.

# The causes of death for men and women aged under 75 years in the UK

Coronary heart disease (CHD) is a major cause of death in the UK among men and women. High levels of cholesterol in your blood increase your risk of developing CHD.

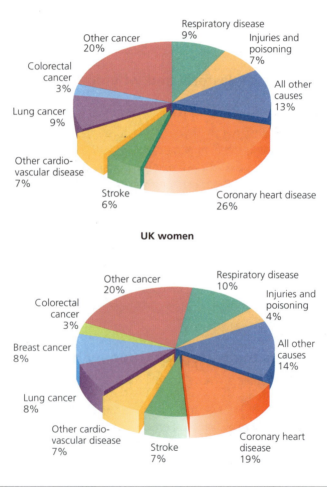

**UK men**

- Respiratory disease 9%
- Injuries and poisoning 7%
- All other causes 13%
- Coronary heart disease 26%
- Stroke 6%
- Other cardio-vascular disease 7%
- Lung cancer 9%
- Colorectal cancer 3%
- Other cancer 20%

**UK women**

- Other cancer 20%
- Respiratory disease 10%
- Injuries and poisoning 4%
- All other causes 14%
- Coronary heart disease 19%
- Stroke 7%
- Other cardio-vascular disease 7%
- Lung cancer 8%
- Breast cancer 8%
- Colorectal cancer 3%

# The incidence of coronary heart disease (CHD) in Europe

Within Europe there are major differences in the incidence of CHD between countries and even within one country. In southern Europe, CHD is generally less common than in northern Europe.

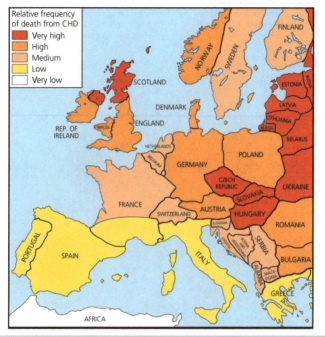

Relative frequency of death from CHD

- Very high
- High
- Medium
- Low
- Very low

The incidence of CHD rose after the Second World War, but is now falling in the UK and North America. However, rates are now rising in developing countries, such as Singapore, Malaysia and eastern Europe.

## The possible consequences of high cholesterol

### Coronary heart disease

Every cell in the body needs oxygen and nutrition to

# The possible clinical consequences of atherosclerosis

Diagram of the body showing the sites affected and the possible clinical consequences of atherosclerosis.

### Coronary heart disease
In CHD the coronary arteries that supply the heart muscle with nutrients become narrowed and the heart muscle becomes starved of the blood that it needs

### Stroke
When a blood vessel supplying vital nutrients to the brain becomes blocked the brain cells that it supplies will die

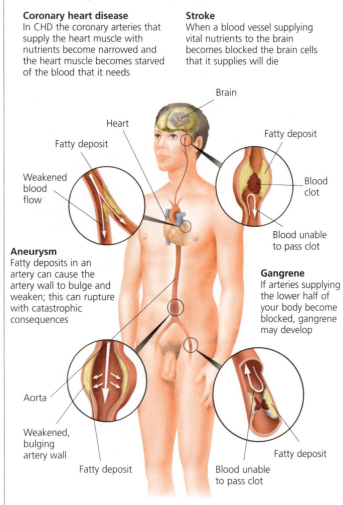

Brain

Heart

Fatty deposit

Weakened blood flow

Fatty deposit

Blood clot

Blood unable to pass clot

### Aneurysm
Fatty deposits in an artery can cause the artery wall to bulge and weaken; this can rupture with catastrophic consequences

### Gangrene
If arteries supplying the lower half of your body become blocked, gangrene may develop

Aorta

Weakened, bulging artery wall

Fatty deposit

Blood unable to pass clot

Fatty deposit

survive, and these essentials are transported around the body in the bloodstream. The blood carries high concentrations of oxygen and 'food' to the cell in the arteries, and carries the waste products of the cell's activity away from the cell in the veins. At the centre of the bloodstream is the heart, which acts as the pump and is responsible for the efficient flow of blood to and from the cells.

Too much cholesterol can lead to narrowing and blockage of arteries. CHD usually results from abnormalities that narrow the arteries supplying blood to your heart – the coronary arteries – hence the name 'coronary heart disease'. Narrowing of these arteries may restrict or completely block the supply of blood to your heart muscle, either of which can cause heart disease.

## Stroke and peripheral vascular disease
This blocking of arteries can also occur in other parts of your circulation. If the blood supply to your brain is affected, a type of stroke may occur, whereas if arteries supplying the lower half of your body become blocked gangrene (blackening and death of skin and muscle) may develop (peripheral vascular disease).

## Aortic aneurysm
These blockages can also weaken the main artery in your body, the aorta, causing a widening or dilatation (called an aneurysm) of its wall, which can rupture with catastrophic consequences.

## Cardiovascular disease
The term 'cardiovascular disease' (CVD) includes CHD, stroke and peripheral vascular disease, together with their complications.

## Atherosclerosis

The process leading to the blockage or weakening of arteries is termed 'atherosclerosis' (sometimes called arteriosclerosis). In the early stages, fatty streaks containing cholesterol develop in arterial walls and these can be found from the late teens onwards.

Fatty streaks are not normal but, in themselves, they don't cause problems and are reversible. However, fatty streaks can develop further and provoke an irreversible reaction in arterial walls. This leads to the laying down of fibrous tissue, rather like a scar, around the cholesterol deposits. These changes don't occur in everyone but they are more common with increasing age.

These changes affect relatively small areas within arteries, and are often raised above the inner surface of arteries, when they are known as plaques. Fibrous plaques are more difficult to reverse than fatty streaks. Plaques can lead to arterial narrowing, so that less blood, and possibly insufficient oxygen, reach certain parts of the body.

Other complications can also occur such as rupturing of a fibrous plaque, leading to a clot forming within the artery (thrombosis). Your artery may become completely blocked when this occurs and, if there is no other blood supply to that area of the body, at least some tissue will die (infarct), causing a heart attack (myocardial infarction), stroke or gangrene.

## Features of coronary heart disease

The features of CHD are caused by changes in arteries supplying blood to the heart and include the following.

### Angina

Chest pain comes on with exertion and improves with

# The process of atherosclerosis

Atherosclerosis, atheroma and hardening of the arteries are all the same thing – the process leading to the blockage or weakening of arteries.

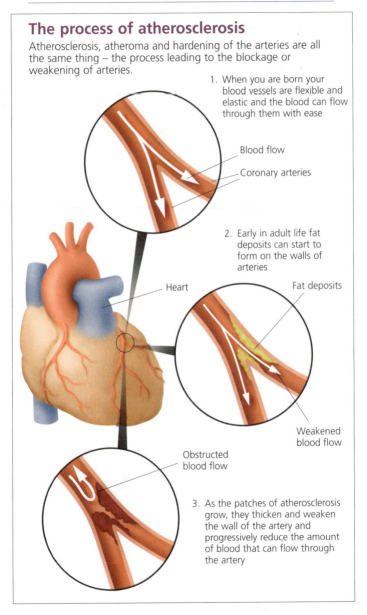

1. When you are born your blood vessels are flexible and elastic and the blood can flow through them with ease

Blood flow

Coronary arteries

2. Early in adult life fat deposits can start to form on the walls of arteries

Heart

Fat deposits

Weakened blood flow

Obstructed blood flow

3. As the patches of atherosclerosis grow, they thicken and weaken the wall of the artery and progressively reduce the amount of blood that can flow through the artery

## How does thrombosis occur?

Thrombosis (formation of blood clots) may be triggered by damage to the lining of a blood vessel. The resulting blood clot may then obstruct the flow of blood through the vessel.

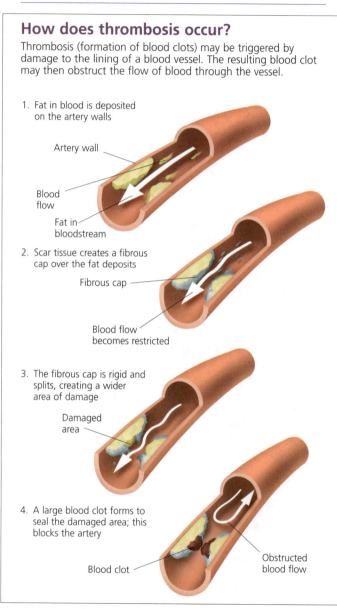

1. Fat in blood is deposited on the artery walls

   Artery wall

   Blood flow

   Fat in bloodstream

2. Scar tissue creates a fibrous cap over the fat deposits

   Fibrous cap

   Blood flow becomes restricted

3. The fibrous cap is rigid and splits, creating a wider area of damage

   Damaged area

4. A large blood clot forms to seal the damaged area; this blocks the artery

   Blood clot

   Obstructed blood flow

rest. Angina is caused by partial blockage of an artery so that insufficient oxygen-rich blood reaches the heart muscle when its requirements increase.

## Myocardial infarction
Severe chest pain occurs when part of the heart muscle dies. This usually results from total blockage of an artery so that no blood reaches the affected tissues.

## Arrhythmia
Abnormal heart rhythm can occur as a result of damage to the heart and may be detectable as palpitations.

## Heart failure
This is a weakening of the pumping action of the heart, and can lead to a build-up of fluid in the body with symptoms such as breathlessness and swollen ankles.

# Risk factors for coronary heart disease
Risk factors are characteristics associated with increased incidence of a disease. You can reduce the likelihood of suffering from CHD by reducing your exposure to 'modifiable' risk factors (for example, stop smoking, lose excess weight). There are some, such as age and gender, that cannot be changed (non-modifiable).

## Non-modifiable risk factors (can't be changed)
Risk factors that you can't change include:

- pre-existing factors
- CHD
- age

| Risk factors for coronary heart disease | |
| --- | --- |
| Non-modifiable risk factors (can't be changed) | Modifiable risk factors (can be changed) |
| • Existing CHD<br>• Age<br>• Family history of CHD<br>• Being male<br>• Ethnic factors | • High blood cholesterol levels<br>• Cigarette smoking<br>• Hypertension<br>• Diabetes mellitus<br>• Obesity<br>• Poor diet<br>• Lack of exercise<br>• Abnormal blood clotting |

• family history of CHD
• male gender.

The risk of having a heart attack is much higher in people who already have CHD than in those without CHD, with the risk increasing nearly three times in those with angina and six times after a previous heart attack.

Heart attacks are more common in older than in young people and also when there is a family history of heart disease. Men are at risk of developing heart disease earlier in life than women. We cannot change our parents, biological sex or previous history, and we are not able to stop the march of time.

CHD is more common in people from the Indian subcontinent living in the UK than in white British people. This ethnic factor is not fully understood, but seems to be partly the result of an increased tendency

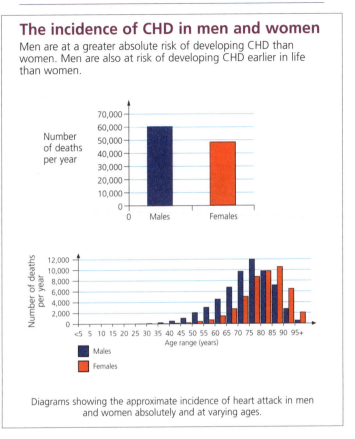

## The incidence of CHD in men and women

Men are at a greater absolute risk of developing CHD than women. Men are also at risk of developing CHD earlier in life than women.

Number of deaths per year

Males   Females

Number of deaths per year

Age range (years)

Males
Females

Diagrams showing the approximate incidence of heart attack in men and women absolutely and at varying ages.

to develop diabetes. CHD incidence is low in those of Chinese origin.

Although you cannot change non-modifiable risk factors, your level of risk from CHD is reduced if your modifiable risk factors are improved. Thus, if you have already had a heart attack and have a raised cholesterol level, you will probably have fewer further heart attacks and live longer if you reduce your fat intake (see page 80).

## Risk factors for coronary heart disease (CHD)

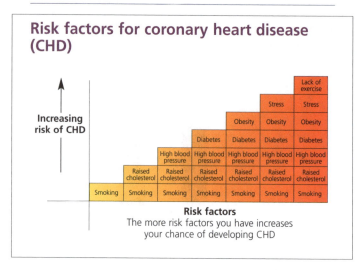

**Increasing risk of CHD**

| | | | | | | Lack of exercise |
| | | | | | Stress | Stress |
| | | | | Obesity | Obesity | Obesity |
| | | | Diabetes | Diabetes | Diabetes | Diabetes |
| | | High blood pressure | High blood pressure | High blood pressure | High blood pressure | High blood pressure |
| | Raised cholesterol | Raised cholesterol | Raised cholesterol | Raised cholesterol | Raised cholesterol | Raised cholesterol |
| Smoking | Smoking | Smoking | Smoking | Smoking | Smoking | Smoking |

**Risk factors**

The more risk factors you have increases your chance of developing CHD

## Modifiable risk factors (can be changed)
### High blood cholesterol, high blood pressure and smoking

High blood cholesterol levels (hypercholesterolaemia), cigarette smoking and high blood pressure (hypertension) are all associated with an increased risk of heart disease.

If you have one of these factors, your risk of developing CHD is increased by two and a half to four times. If you have more than one risk factor, the risk multiplies. The risk for someone with hypertension who smokes cigarettes and has a high blood cholesterol level is about 30 times higher than for a non-smoker with normal blood pressure and a low cholesterol level.

This increased risk can be reduced significantly by lowering high blood pressure, reducing blood cholesterol and stopping smoking. Hypertension and smoking do not affect cholesterol levels but interact with cholesterol in damaging arteries.

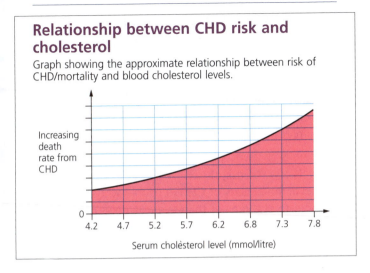

## Relationship between CHD risk and cholesterol

Graph showing the approximate relationship between risk of CHD/mortality and blood cholesterol levels.

Increasing death rate from CHD

Serum cholesterol level (mmol/litre)

4.2  4.7  5.2  5.7  6.2  6.8  7.3  7.8

## Diabetes

People with both type 1 and type 2 diabetes mellitus have a higher incidence of arterial disease, and are more likely to suffer a heart attack or stroke than someone without diabetes. Careful treatment of diabetes will reduce this risk, although it is also important to address any other CHD risk factors that are present. For example, abnormal blood fat levels and hypertension are more common in people with diabetes than in the non-diabetic population (see page 45).

## Weight

Obesity increases the risk of CHD, particularly if fat is deposited around the abdomen rather than the shoulders and thighs. Lifestyle factors such as a diet rich in fat and lack of exercise are also important. A further risk factor is high blood levels of specific proteins that promote clotting – these can be detected through blood tests.

# Do high blood cholesterol levels cause CHD?

The short answer is yes, for the following reasons:

- People develop CHD whereas it is not seen in other animals under natural conditions, and people have higher cholesterol levels than other animals. If cholesterol levels are artificially raised in laboratory animals they can develop atherosclerosis.

- There is an association between blood cholesterol levels and the risk of CHD. The graph on page 13 shows more cases of CHD in people whose blood cholesterol is greater than five millimoles of cholesterol per litre of blood (usually shortened to mmol/l; a millimole is a way of quantifying a very small amount of a substance).

- Some people are born with a genetic abnormality in the way that their body handles cholesterol. There are several such conditions, of which the most common is familial hypercholesterolaemia (familial means it runs in families). Patients with this condition often have blood cholesterol levels that are two or three times higher than normal. In general, they have a much greater risk of developing CHD than those without the condition (see page 43).

- Effective treatment of hypercholesterolaemia with drugs called statins reduces the incidence of CHD. This means that there are fewer heart attacks and a slower progression of the changes in the arteries. This improves life expectancy and reduces the need for an operation called a coronary artery bypass graft.

Taking all these factors together, there is little doubt that high blood cholesterol levels cause heart disease.

## How do strokes occur?

The most common cause of a stroke is a thrombosis – when a blood vessel supplying the brain becomes blocked with a blood clot. The second most common cause of a stroke is a brain haemorrhage, of which there are two types; both involve a blood vessel bursting inside the head.

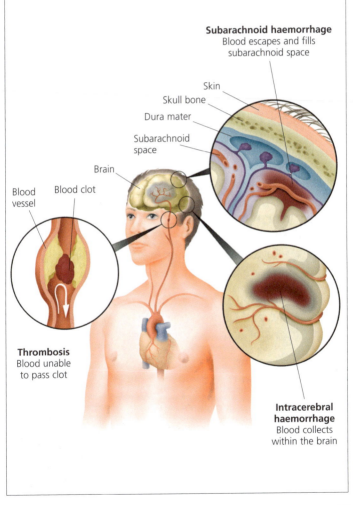

**Subarachnoid haemorrhage**
Blood escapes and fills subarachnoid space

Skin

Skull bone

Dura mater

Subarachnoid space

Brain

Blood vessel

Blood clot

**Thrombosis**
Blood unable to pass clot

**Intracerebral haemorrhage**
Blood collects within the brain

## Risk factors for stroke

There are two main types of stroke, one caused by bleeding (haemorrhage) in or around the brain, and the other caused by blockage of an artery supplying blood to the brain (ischaemic stroke). The changes in the arteries that cause ischaemic stroke are similar to those causing CHD and many of the risk factors are the same, including increasing age, high blood pressure, pre-existing arterial disease and smoking. Treatment with statins reduces the numbers of this type of stroke.

There are some differences, however. If you have a high alcohol intake your risk of stroke is increased, and blood cholesterol levels are a weaker risk factor for ischaemic stroke than for CHD.

### KEY POINTS

- CHD and stroke result from disease in artery walls

- A number of factors increase the likelihood of developing CHD and other forms of cardiovascular disease

- Cholesterol is deposited in diseased arteries and can lead to their narrowing

- High blood cholesterol levels are a risk factor for heart disease and stroke

- Controlling high blood cholesterol levels reduces the risk of cardiovascular disease

# Lipids important to the body

## What are lipids?

Cholesterol is a type of lipid (fat). Lipids are substances that do not dissolve in water but are soluble in organic solvents such as chloroform or dry cleaning fluids. Other important types of lipid include triglycerides and fatty acids.

Lipids have several important roles in the body, providing:

- a source and store of energy
- an important part of the membrane surrounding every body cell
- the basic building blocks from which several hormones (chemical messengers) and bile acids (digestive juices) are made
- components of the nervous system.

## All about cholesterol
### The importance of cholesterol

Some cholesterol comes from your food, but most is made in your body, mainly in your liver, from the saturated fats (animal and dairy fat) that you eat.

## Cell structures

Cholesterol occurs in every cell of your body and forms a vital part of the membrane that surrounds each cell, preventing cells from being too leaky.

## Hormones

Cholesterol is also the basis for many hormones, essential for the regulation of growth and the way your body works on a day-to-day basis. Hormones made using cholesterol include the following.

## Oestrogens and progestogens

These hormones are produced by the ovaries and are responsible for female sexual characteristics and the menstrual cycle.

## Testosterone

This hormone is produced by the testes and is responsible for male sexual characteristics and sperm production.

## Cortisol

Cortisol is produced by the adrenal glands (there is one on the top of each kidney). Cortisol regulates your body's response to stress.

## Aldosterone

Like cortisol, aldosterone is produced by the adrenal glands. Its main function is to ensure that the levels of salt and potassium in the body are normal.

## 1,25-Dihydroxycholecalciferol, the active form of vitamin D

Vitamin D is present in a well-balanced diet and is also produced in your skin on exposure to sunlight,

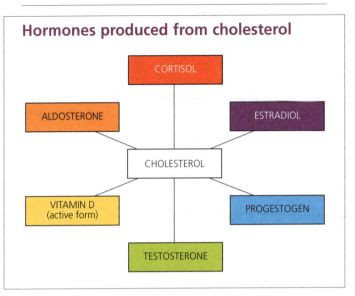

## Hormones produced from cholesterol

CORTISOL

ALDOSTERONE

ESTRADIOL

CHOLESTEROL

VITAMIN D (active form)

PROGESTOGEN

TESTOSTERONE

particularly in summer months. Vitamin D is modified by your liver and kidneys to produce a hormone, 1,25-dihydroxycholecalciferol. This controls calcium absorption from your gut, as well as normal bone development and health. Vitamin D deficiency in childhood causes rickets, whereas deficiency in adults leads to softening of the bones (osteomalacia).

## Digestion

Bile acids are also made from cholesterol in the liver and act like detergents in your gut, dissolving fat from your food. This is necessary for the normal digestion and absorption of lipids and fat-soluble vitamins (A, D, E and K). If bile acids don't reach your gut from the gallbladder, where they are stored, fat is not digested properly – the result is diarrhoea, and the fat is lost in pale, very smelly stools.

Although it is clear that too much cholesterol can cause heart disease, it would be impossible to survive without it.

### Chemical structure of cholesterol
Cholesterol has a very different structure to triglycerides (see page 22), although both are virtually insoluble in water. Cholesterol consists of carbon molecules linked in a series of rings; substances with this type of structure are termed 'sterols'.

## All about triglycerides
### The importance of triglycerides
Your body's fat stores contain triglycerides and these act as an important source of energy. Some are made in your body, whereas others come from your food.

### Structure of cholesterol
Simplified molecular structure of cholesterol.

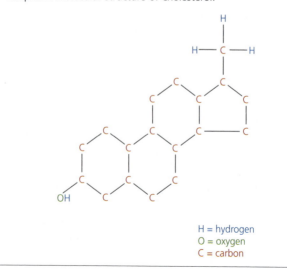

H = hydrogen
O = oxygen
C = carbon

After a meal, small amounts of sugar (glucose) are stored in your liver and muscle as larger molecules called glycogen (molecules are the smallest identifiable units of a substance).

Glycogen can supply short-term energy needs between meals or during short bursts of physical activity, such as sprinting. This is because it can make energy available very rapidly by breaking down to glucose. However, glycogen provides less than half the calories per gram that can come from fat stored as triglycerides.

In addition, glycogen is stored surrounded by water whereas triglycerides are not. You would therefore be considerably heavier if all your energy stores were in the form of glycogen (a 70-kilogram [kg] man would be 210 kg!).

Triglycerides, through the fatty acids that they contain, provide most of your body's energy needs when you have not eaten for several hours, and can also supply your energy needs directly during prolonged exercise, such as running any distance greater than 400 metres.

If the process of using fatty acids to provide energy needs is disturbed in any way, you get hypoglycaemia (low blood sugar levels), particularly between meals.

As well as providing a vital source of energy, triglycerides help to make food palatable. It is extremely difficult to tolerate for very long a diet that includes less than 25 grams of fat per day.

## Chemical structure of triglycerides

Triglycerides are composed of three fatty acids linked together by a small molecule called glycerol.

## Structure of a triglyceride and a fatty acid

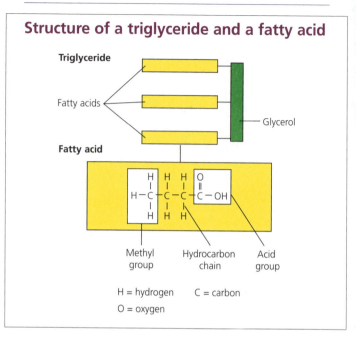

H = hydrogen     C = carbon
O = oxygen

## All about fatty acids

Fatty acids consist of long chains of carbon atoms linked together. There are two main types of fatty acids: saturated and unsaturated. Unsaturated fats can be either monounsaturated or polyunsaturated.

## Saturated fatty acids

All the carbon atoms in the chains are linked by single chemical bonds; this type of fatty acid is found in large amounts in the triglycerides present in animal fat.

## Monounsaturated fatty acids

All the links between carbon atoms in the chains are saturated bonds except for one that is unsaturated (a double bond). These occur in vegetable oils, such as olive oil and rapeseed oil.

## Polyunsaturated fatty acids

More of the links between carbon atoms in the chain are unsaturated – as many as five or more. Fish oils are a particularly rich source of polyunsaturated fatty acids of a type sometimes called omega-3 fatty acids. Polyunsaturated fatty acids are also found in plant oils, such as sunflower oil.

## How do fatty acids affect health?

The type of fatty acids in your diet affects your health. People with a relatively high intake of olive oil or fish

---

## Structures of fatty acids

Simplified molecular structure of a saturated, monounsaturated and polyunsaturated fatty acid.

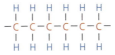

A saturated fatty acid

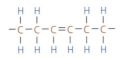

A monounsaturated fatty acid

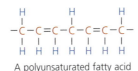

H = hydrogen
C = carbon

A polyunsaturated fatty acid

(polyunsaturated fatty acids) have a lower incidence of heart disease than those who have a relatively high intake of saturated fat (see page 84).

Saturated fatty acids raise blood cholesterol levels, whereas monounsaturated fatty acids do not affect blood cholesterol levels. The main effect of polyunsaturated fatty acids on blood lipids is to lower serum triglyceride concentrations, but they do not affect cholesterol.

## Other lipids

Several other lipids are also found in your body. Some are vital components of your brain. An important group includes phospholipids, which resemble triglycerides in structure – the main difference is that one of the fatty acid groups is replaced by one that contains phosphorus. This alters the properties of the molecule because half of its structure is soluble in fat whereas the other dissolves in water. These dual solubility properties allow phospholipids to act as detergents and, together with special proteins, phospholipids are able to interact with cholesterol and triglycerides to form packages of lipids that are stable in water (lipoproteins, see page 26).

**KEY POINTS**

■ Triglycerides (found in animal and dairy fats) are the main form of energy store in your body

■ Cholesterol is a lipid (fat) and does not dissolve in water

■ Cholesterol is essential for normal cell structure

■ Several vital hormones are made from cholesterol

# Bad cholesterol and good cholesterol

## Where does cholesterol come from?

The cholesterol in your body comes from two sources: your diet and what you make yourself. Typically, around seven times more cholesterol is made in your body from dietary saturated fats (animal and dairy fat) than is absorbed as cholesterol from your food.

Most cholesterol is made in your liver, but small amounts are also made in almost all other cells in the body, particularly those found in the intestines, adrenal cortex and skin. Your liver can provide all the cholesterol that your body needs, so cholesterol is not an essential part of your diet.

Dietary cholesterol is absorbed from your small intestines, and travels in the blood to your liver, where it mixes with cholesterol produced in the liver itself. Cholesterol from these two sources then travels to other body tissues where it is needed to make cell membranes, and to act as a building block for making steroid hormones or vitamin D.

## The role of lipoproteins

As cholesterol does not dissolve in blood serum, which

is mostly water, it is first stabilised for transportation. This is done by packaging it in particles called lipoproteins. Lipoproteins are made up of:

- cholesterol and triglycerides (which both need to be transported around the body)
- specialised proteins called apolipoproteins (sometimes shortened to apoproteins or apos)
- phospholipids.

The phospholipids act as detergents which dissolve fats, whereas the proteins help to make the particles stable. It is in this form that cholesterol and triglycerides are transported around the body.

There are five main types of plasma lipoprotein, all of which have slightly different functions and which get their names from their relative density (size and weight) – see the box on page 28.

The two types that are most important for cholesterol transport are low-density lipoprotein (LDL) and high-density lipoprotein (HDL). Most of the cholesterol in blood is in LDL particles – there are more HDL particles than LDL, but HDL particles contain relatively more protein and less cholesterol in each particle.

## Cholesterol transport around the body
### To body tissues

The liver is the central organ for handling cholesterol. It makes and prepares cholesterol for transport to other organs. Cholesterol and triglycerides are packaged together into very-low-density lipoprotein (VLDL) particles. These particles reach the bloodstream and are carried around your body.

## Lipoproteins and their functions

There are five main types of lipoprotein, all of which have slightly different functions.

### Chylomicrons
Made in the small intestine; carry dietary fatty acids directly from the gut to the liver and peripheral tissues where it will be used or stored as fuel

### Very-low-density lipoproteins (VLDLs)
Made in the liver; carry excess fatty acids from the liver to adipose tissue (fat tissue), where free fatty acids are released and taken up by fat cells for storage

### Intermediate-density lipoproteins (IDLs)
Made from VLDLs after free fatty acids are released; taken up by the liver and converted into LDL particles

### Low-density lipoproteins (LDLs)
The main carrier of cholesterol, taking it to peripheral tissues with excess returning to the liver

### High-density lipoproteins (HDLs)
Made in the liver and intestines; collect cholesterol from cell membranes in peripheral tissues and transport it back to the liver for processing (reverse cholesterol transport)

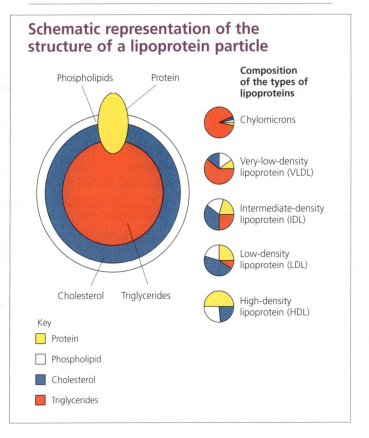

## Schematic representation of the structure of a lipoprotein particle

Phospholipids    Protein

Cholesterol    Triglycerides

**Composition of the types of lipoproteins**

Chylomicrons

Very-low-density lipoprotein (VLDL)

Intermediate-density lipoprotein (IDL)

Low-density lipoprotein (LDL)

High-density lipoprotein (HDL)

Key

☐ Protein

☐ Phospholipid

☐ Cholesterol

☐ Triglycerides

The triglycerides are removed as VLDL passes through organs, and their fatty acids are used as energy for muscles or stored to create energy reserves in adipose (fat) tissue. The VLDL particles become smaller as triglycerides are removed and change into LDLs. As triglycerides have been removed, LDLs are rich in cholesterol.

## Locks and keys

The purpose of LDL is to deliver cholesterol to body tissues. Tissues have small pits in their cell walls (LDL receptors), which can be thought of as locks. LDL particles have a special protein on their surface called apoprotein B (or apoB). This is the key that opens the lock of the cell receptors. When the key fits into the lock, the door opens and LDL particles pass into the cell.

Once inside, LDL particles dissolve, releasing the cholesterol that they contain, thus supplying the cells' needs. Most of the cells' cholesterol requirements are met in this way, although cells can also manufacture cholesterol when LDL particles cannot get into cells (for example, in familial hypercholesterolaemia – see page 38).

## From body tissues

Cholesterol is continually removed from cells in high-density lipoproteins (HDLs), which take cholesterol from cells to the liver; this then excretes it in the bile. Thus, as well as producing cholesterol, the liver can also remove cholesterol from the blood. Excess cholesterol from cells can be removed from the body by this mechanism.

## Lipoproteins and CVD

LDL is sometimes thought of as containing bad cholesterol whereas HDL is regarded as carrying good cholesterol. This is because of the different associations between CVD (cardiovascular disease) and blood levels of these lipoproteins.

## LDLs and CVD

The link between high blood cholesterol levels and CVD was outlined on page 12, and it is the cholesterol

## How cholesterol is transported to the tissues of the body

VLDL particles pass through capillary walls into the surrounding tissues, releasing triglyceride and so becoming LDLs.

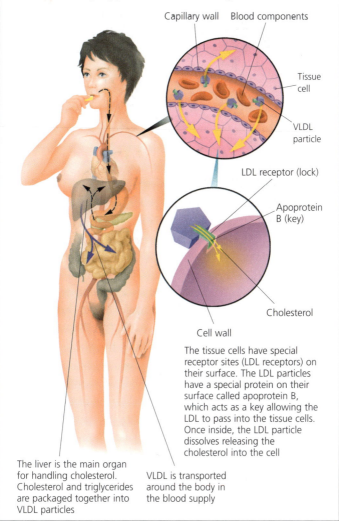

Capillary wall

Blood components

Tissue cell

VLDL particle

LDL receptor (lock)

Apoprotein B (key)

Cholesterol

Cell wall

The tissue cells have special receptor sites (LDL receptors) on their surface. The LDL particles have a special protein on their surface called apoprotein B, which acts as a key allowing the LDL to pass into the tissue cells. Once inside, the LDL particle dissolves releasing the cholesterol into the cell

The liver is the main organ for handling cholesterol. Cholesterol and triglycerides are packaged together into VLDL particles

VLDL is transported around the body in the blood supply

## How cholesterol is removed from the tissues of the body

Cholesterol is continually removed from cells in HDL which takes the cholesterol back to the liver where it is excreted in the bile.

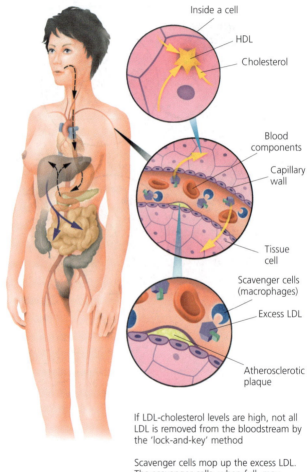

Inside a cell

HDL

Cholesterol

Blood components

Capillary wall

Tissue cell

Scavenger cells (macrophages)

Excess LDL

Atherosclerotic plaque

If LDL-cholesterol levels are high, not all LDL is removed from the bloodstream by the 'lock-and-key' method

Scavenger cells mop up the excess LDL. The scavenger cells, when full, may deposit on the walls of blood vessels, starting the process of arterial disease

## Bad cholesterol (LDL) versus good cholesterol (HDL)

Low-density lipoprotein (LDL) is sometimes thought of as containing bad cholesterol, whereas high-density lipoprotein (HDL) is regarded as carrying good cholesterol.

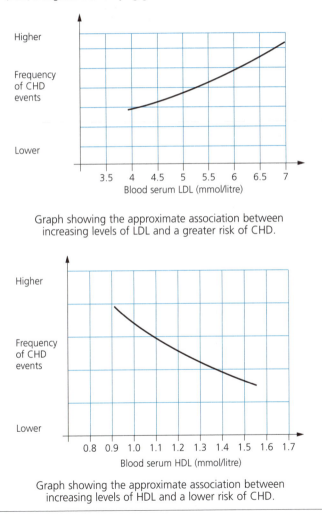

Graph showing the approximate association between increasing levels of LDL and a greater risk of CHD.

Graph showing the approximate association between increasing levels of HDL and a lower risk of CHD.

in LDLs that is responsible for causing atherosclerosis. If LDL-cholesterol levels are high, they are not all removed from the blood by the lock-and-key mechanism outlined earlier. LDL particles find their way through artery walls where they are taken up by macrophages.

Macrophages are scavenger cells that mop up excess particles, such as LDLs, as well as micro-organisms and worn-out proteins. When full of cholesterol these scavenger cells start the process that leads to the development of atherosclerotic plaques and arterial disease. Thus, high LDL levels are bad for health.

## HDLs and CVD

Increasingly high blood levels of HDLs are associated with lower risks of developing CVD, hence the view that HDLs contain good cholesterol. The reasons for this are not absolutely clear, but possibly relate to the fact that HDLs remove cholesterol from cells and carry it to the liver. HDLs might therefore prevent cholesterol building up in key sites such as arterial walls, lessening the risk of atherosclerosis.

### HDL and antioxidant activity

A further possibility for the protective effects of HDL is that it has antioxidant activity. Oxidation of LDL is thought to occur before the particles are taken up by macrophages in arterial walls, and there is some evidence that antioxidants may prevent this change occurring in LDL particles, and protect against the development of atherosclerosis. Thus, the protective effect of HDL against CVD could be the result of it preventing oxidation of LDL, rather than removing excess cholesterol from cells. It has also been suggested that HDL protects the cells that line the walls of arteries.

## Triglycerides and CVD

There is more controversy about a link between raised blood triglyceride levels and CVD than there is for cholesterol. The main reason for this is that the results of clinical studies of triglycerides and CVD have been inconsistent. A further complication is that the levels of LDLs and HDLs are usually affected if blood triglycerides are high. Despite uncertainties, the link between high blood levels of triglycerides and CVD is clearer in women than in men and is also seen in diabetes. This is discussed more fully on page 107.

Very high levels of blood triglycerides increase the risk of developing an inflammation of the pancreas, pancreatitis (see page 106).

## KEY POINTS

- Some cholesterol comes from your diet, but most is made in your body – mainly in liver cells

- Cholesterol is carried in your blood around your body in particles called lipoproteins

- High LDL levels are associated with CVD

- High HDL levels seem to protect against CVD

# What causes high blood cholesterol levels?

## What is hypercholesterolaemia?

The term 'hypercholesterolaemia' means high blood cholesterol levels. 'Hyperlipidaemia' is a less specific term that refers to an increase in one or more blood fat levels. As both cholesterol and triglycerides are fats, hyperlipidaemia could be used to indicate raised blood levels of either.

High blood cholesterol levels are caused by two main types of condition: primary and secondary hypercholesterolaemia:

- Primary hypercholesterolaemia results from inherited genetic abnormalities that lead to increased blood cholesterol levels.

- Secondary hypercholesterolaemia is found when a disease produces high blood cholesterol levels as a complication.

It is important for doctors to make this distinction because it affects the treatment. Primary hypercholesterolaemia may require direct treatment, whereas secondary hypercholesterolaemia usually improves on its own if the underlying disease is treated.

## Primary genetic (inherited) causes of hyperlipidaemia
### Familial hypercholesterolaemia

The way in which lipids are transported in the blood and taken up by cells is controlled by a number of proteins, two of which, apoB and the low-density lipoprotein (LDL) receptor, were discussed on pages 27–30. A common genetic cause of hypercholesterolaemia is a defect in the LDL receptors (the 'locks' that allow LDL particles to enter cells), which results in familial hypercholesterolaemia.

A single gene controls LDL receptors in our bodies. We inherit one copy of this gene from our mother and one copy from our father, and both of these copies operate.

### How common is it?

In the UK, about 1 in 500 people has a fault in one of these genes. In some parts of the world it is more common – for example, one per cent (1 in 100) of the Afrikaner population in South Africa have the condition. There is often a strong family history of early coronary heart disease (CHD) in relatives of patients with familial hypercholesterolaemia, sometimes affecting several generations of the family.

### Why are blood cholesterol levels raised?

People with familial hypercholesterolaemia have only

## Causes of hypercholesterolaemia

### Primary (genetic) hypercholesterolaemia

- Single abnormal gene, for example, familial hypercholesterolaemia
- Minor variations in several genes combined with a high-fat diet (polygenic hypercholesterolaemia)
- Familial combined hyperlipidaemia (raised cholesterol and triglyceride levels)
- Rare genetic disorders

### Secondary hypercholesterolaemia

- Diabetes mellitus
- Obesity
- Alcohol abuse
- Hypothyroidism (underactive thyroid gland)
- Liver disease
- Kidney disease
- Drugs, for example, Roaccutane used to treat severe acne, thiazide diuretics used to treat fluid retention or high blood pressure, some beta-blocking drugs used to treat high blood pressure or angina

half the usual number of normal LDL receptors. As a result, fewer LDL particles are taken up by body cells, so there are more in the blood than normal. These excess LDL particles, together with the cholesterol that they contain, are taken up by scavenger cells and find their way into the walls of arteries where they build up to produce fatty streaks and atherosclerosis.

The risk of CHD developing in people with familial hypercholesterolaemia is significantly higher than in those without the condition. About 50 per cent of men with this condition will die before the age of 60 years unless their high blood cholesterol levels are treated effectively with cholesterol-lowering drugs, together with dietary and lifestyle changes. But before you can be treated, the condition must be diagnosed.

## Diagnosing hypercholesterolaemia

Sometimes there are signs that suggest that hyper-cholesterolaemia may be present. These include tendon xanthomas, xanthelasmas and corneal arcus.

## Tendon xanthomas

These are swellings on the tendons of muscles, typically the Achilles' heel, on the backs of the hands or on the elbows. They are caused by deposits of cholesterol and strongly suggest that familial hypercholesterolaemia may be present. They may weaken the tendons, which can then snap when they are being strained – for example, during vigorous physical exercise.

## Xanthelasmas

These are cholesterol deposits in the skin around the eye.

## Corneal arcus

This is a white ring found in the outer part of the cornea of the eye. It can appear as we grow older and, under these circumstances, has little significance. However, it is found at a younger age (in the 30s and 40s) in patients with familial hypercholesterolaemia and may be picked up by an optician during a routine eye test.

## The possible signs of hypercholesterolaemia

Sometimes there are signs which suggest that hypercholesterol-aemia may be present. These include tendon xanthomas, xanthelasmas and corneal arcus.

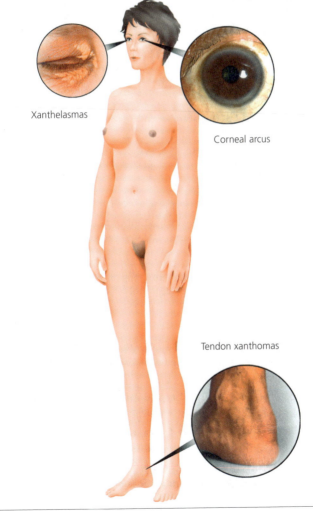

Xanthelasmas

Corneal arcus

Tendon xanthomas

## Criteria for the diagnosis of familial hypercholesterolaemia

### Definite familial hypercholesterolaemia

- Blood cholesterol level above 6.7 millimoles per litre (mmol/l) in children or 7.5 mmol/l in adults

*plus*

- Tendon xanthomas in the patient or in a close relative

### Possible familial hypercholesterolaemia

- Blood cholesterol level above 6.7 mmol/l in children or 7.5 mmol/l in adults

*plus*

- Family history of a heart attack below the age of 50 in a grandparent, uncle, aunt or cousin, or below the age of 60 years in a parent, brother or sister

*or*

- Family history of blood cholesterol levels above 7.5 mmol/l in a close relative

Although xanthelasmas and corneal arcus occur with increased frequency in familial hypercholesterolaemia, they also occur in patients with normal blood cholesterol levels and in those with hypercholesterolaemia from other causes. If found, they indicate that the blood cholesterol levels should be measured (see page 60), although these levels will often be normal.

Sometimes there are no clues that familial hypercholesterolaemia may be present before a heart attack occurs.

The diagnosis of familial hypercholesterolaemia depends on a number of criteria (see the box above).

## Inheriting familial hypercholesterolaemia

If you have familial hypercholesterolaemia, you have a 50:50 chance of passing it on to any children that you may have. This is because each child will hopefully inherit a normal gene from your partner and has a 50 per cent chance of inheriting the abnormal gene from you.

Very rarely, both parents have the condition. As the incidence of familial hypercholesterolaemia is 1 in 500 in the UK, the chances of this happening are 1 in $500^2$ – that is, 1 in 250,000. In this case, each parent has one normal and one abnormal gene. Therefore, if they have four children the chances are that one child will be normal, two children will have one abnormal gene (and will therefore have the more common form of familial hypercholesterolaemia) and one child will inherit two abnormal genes.

Two abnormal genes cause a much more severe form of familial hypercholesterolaemia than inheriting just one abnormal gene, and CHD is more severe and occurs earlier, often in the early teens.

There is little chance of someone with two abnormal genes reaching middle age without very extensive treatment, such as a type of dialysis treatment (to remove excess fats from the blood) or a liver transplantation to provide normal LDL receptors. It is fortunate that this very severe form of the disease is very rare.

## Polygenic hypercholesterolaemia

Polygenic hypercholesterolaemia is more common than familial hypercholesterolaemia, affecting around one in five people. Rather than an abnormality of a single gene, small variations occur in several genes that regulate how the body deals with cholesterol. This results in hypercholesterolaemia if people with the condition eat food that is relatively high in fat, particularly saturated fat – typical behaviour in this country, other northern European countries and the USA.

This type of hypercholesterolaemia usually responds to reducing saturated fat intake, and people with this condition usually show a more satisfactory response to diet and lifestyle changes than those with familial hypercholesterolaemia.

The risk of CHD is increased two- to threefold in polygenic hypercholesterolaemia, although the increased risk is not as high as in familial hypercholesterolaemia. The pattern of inheritance is less clear and there may be no history of early CHD in relatives. Xanthelasmas and premature corneal arcus may occur, but not tendon xanthomas.

## Familial combined hyperlipidaemia

When blood levels of both cholesterol and triglycerides are increased it is known as combined hyperlipidaemia or, if it is hereditary, familial combined hyperlipidaemia. Raised blood triglyceride levels may also occur in both polygenic and familial hypercholesterolaemia, but is usually a minor finding in these conditions, increases in triglycerides being modest.

Combined hyperlipidaemia occurs when LDL particles contain some triglyceride, or when the number of very-low-density lipoprotein (VLDL) particles (which contain more triglyceride than LDL) is increased.

In familial combined hyperlipidaemia, the pattern of blood fat levels may vary between family members, or even in the same patient at different times. Thus, both blood cholesterol and triglyceride levels may be raised or just blood cholesterol. The features are similar to those seen in polygenic hypercholesterolaemia.

### Other inherited forms of hyperlipidaemia

There are other inherited causes of hyperlipidaemia, some of which affect blood triglyceride levels more than cholesterol, and so hypertriglyceridaemia can be the predominant abnormality (see page 106).

## Secondary hyperlipidaemia

Raised blood cholesterol and/or triglyceride levels may be found in a number of conditions outlined in the box on page 39. The abnormal blood lipids occur as a result of the disease or behaviour, rather than an underlying abnormality in body fats.

### Diabetes mellitus

Diabetes mellitus is often thought of as a disease affecting just the way that the body handles glucose. However, disturbances of other body processes are extremely common in diabetes, and hyperlipidaemia is frequently present, particularly in the adult form of the disease (type 2 diabetes mellitus).

The most characteristic lipid changes are high blood triglyceride levels and low levels of cholesterol in HDL particles (HDL-cholesterol). Occasionally, total cholesterol is elevated. Rarely, more significant changes in blood triglyceride levels occur, particularly if diabetes is poorly controlled (see page 106).

The blood lipid levels usually improve with effective management of blood glucose levels, but the risk of CHD and other forms of arterial disease is very high in

# The risk of CHD increases in overweight people

The increased risk occurs mainly from the 'android' pattern of obesity. The 'gynaecoid' pattern has a lesser effect on the risk of CHD.

Gynaecoid pattern of obesity – affects mainly shoulders and buttocks; more common in women

Android pattern of obesity – produces an enlarged waist; more common in men

this condition, being similar to that in patients with existing CHD. For this reason, abnormalities of blood lipid levels are often treated with drugs if they don't respond to diet and medication to control the diabetes. Many people with type 2 diabetes are overweight, and both the diabetes and blood lipid abnormalities can improve if they lose weight.

## Obesity

Two patterns of obesity are recognised, one mostly affecting the shoulders and buttocks (gynaecoid pattern, more common in women), and the other producing an enlarged waist (android pattern, more common in men).

The risk of CHD is doubled in those who are 50 per cent overweight, this increased risk resulting mainly from the android pattern of obesity. The reason is poorly understood but thought to relate to two factors: a greater incidence of high blood pressure and an abnormality in the way that the body handles dietary fats. Abnormalities of blood fats occur in the android pattern, for example, with changes resembling those seen in diabetes mellitus (raised triglyceride and low HDL-cholesterol levels). Blood fats are usually normal in the gynaecoid pattern, and it has a lesser effect on the risk of CHD.

Abnormal blood fat levels respond to weight reduction, similar to the situation in diabetes. However, many obese patients find this very difficult to achieve.

## Alcohol abuse

Moderate alcohol intake seems to protect against CHD and has beneficial effects on blood lipids (see page 78). However, excess alcohol intake can lead to large increases in blood lipids, particularly triglycerides, because liver cells stop their normal processing of dietary fats in order to detoxify the alcohol, which is a powerful cell poison.

Very rarely, triglyceride levels may increase by 80 to 100 times. Total cholesterol levels may also be raised (see page 106).

The hyperlipidaemia of excess alcohol intake responds to reduced consumption of alcohol.

### Hypothyroidism

Hypercholesterolaemia is common when the thyroid gland is underactive (hypothyroidism), to such an extent that, before reliable measurements of thyroid hormone levels became available, blood cholesterol concentrations were used as a test of how well the thyroid gland was working.

## Hypercholesterolaemia and hypothyroidism

Hypercholesterolaemia is common when the thyroid gland is underactive (hypothyroidism). If hypothyroidism is treated, abnormal cholesterol levels will usually improve.

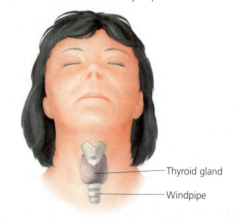

Thyroid gland

Windpipe

If hypothyroidism is treated with thyroid hormone replacement, abnormal cholesterol levels usually improve, although doctors often check the levels again once the thyroid condition has been controlled. This is because both thyroid problems and hypercholesterol-aemia are relatively common and the two conditions are not always related.

### Liver and kidney disease

Both liver and kidney (renal) disease can produce abnormal blood fat levels. Hypercholesterolaemia is common if the outflow of bile from the liver is impaired as a result of a blockage in the bile duct. This is because excess cholesterol is removed from the body in the bile.

In some types of renal disease the production of LDL particles is increased, whereas in others the removal of triglycerides from the blood is reduced. These changes may partly explain the increased risk of CHD that occurs in people with kidney failure.

### Drugs

Some drugs can raise blood lipids, usually affecting triglycerides more than cholesterol. These increases are often quite high, such as the hypertriglyceridaemia seen occasionally with Roaccutane, a drug used to treat acne.

Interestingly, some drugs used to treat heart disease can also lead to hyperlipidaemia, such as thiazide diuretics ('water tablets', also used to treat high blood pressure) and beta-blocking agents (used mainly in the treatment of high blood pressure or angina). This doesn't mean that the use of these drugs is inappropriate – the benefit may be greater than any increased risk from lipids. An example of this is the use of thiazide diuretics in the treatment of high blood pressure. Such drugs can cause slight increases in blood lipid levels, but the advantage resulting from the lowering of blood pressure, leading to a lower incidence of stroke, outweighs the negative effect on lipids.

## KEY POINTS

- Hypercholesterolaemia may be caused by an inherited abnormality

- Raised blood triglyceride levels may accompany hypercholesterolaemia

- Hyperlipidaemia may result from other diseases such as diabetes or an underactive thyroid gland

# How is hyper-cholesterolaemia diagnosed?

Findings such as tendon xanthomas, xanthelasmas or early corneal arcus (see page 40) may suggest that hypercholesterolaemia is present, but the only way to be sure is to take a blood sample and measure blood cholesterol levels.

## What is high?

The average total cholesterol level in blood in the UK is around 5.2 millimoles per litre (mmol/l). About 20 per cent of people have a level above 6.5 mmol/l.

The more your cholesterol level is above average, the higher your risk of cardiovascular disease (CVD). What cholesterol level is regarded as 'high' is determined by the association between the risk of CVD and blood cholesterol levels (see page 12).

The risk of CVD doubles as the blood cholesterol concentration increases from 5.2 mmol/l (expressed as 200 mg/100 ml in America) to 6.5 mmol/l (250 mg/100 ml) and is about three times higher if the cholesterol level is 7.8 mmol/l (300 mg/100 ml).

# What should I expect my cholesterol level to be?

The average total cholesterol level in blood in the UK is around 5.2 millimoles per litre. This average value conceals a good deal of variability as the first graph below shows. Your gender and age also have a significant influence (see second graph).

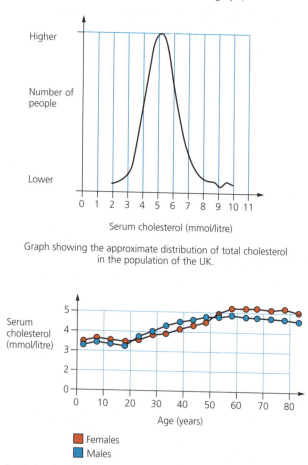

Graph showing the approximate distribution of total cholesterol in the population of the UK.

Graph showing the approximate differences in average blood cholesterol by age and gender in the UK.

## What should I expect my cholesterol level to be? (contd)

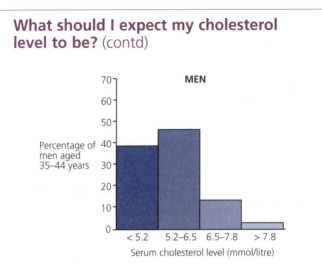

Diagram showing the approximate distribution of total cholesterol in men aged 35–44 years.

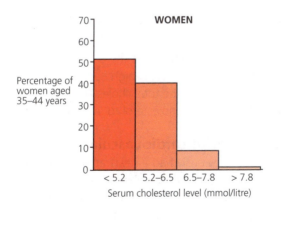

Diagram showing the approximate distribution of total cholesterol in women aged 35–44 years.

So the relative risk of dying from a heart attack is doubled if your total cholesterol is 6.5 mmol/l rather than 5.2 mmol/l. This sounds a very significant increase in risk, although it is important to understand this in absolute as well as in relative terms.

For example, if no other risk factors are present, a young adult with a cholesterol level of 5.2 mmol/l has a very small risk of dying from CVD (0.08 per cent per year or 1 in 1,250). This increases to 0.16 per cent (1 in 625) if the cholesterol level is 6.5 mmol/l. Although the risk has doubled, it still remains very small, but relatively high compared with the person's peers. It increases again to 0.24 per cent (1 in 417) if the cholesterol level is 7.8 mmol/l.

In terms of these risks, it is clearly desirable to have a cholesterol level of less than 5 mmol/l. People with higher levels would almost certainly benefit from diet and lifestyle changes aimed at reducing cholesterol.

A blood total cholesterol level of 6.5 mmol/l or more is considered 'high', although the absolute risk at this level is not considered high enough to require treatment with drugs unless other risk factors, such as high blood pressure and smoking, are present and the overall risk of CVD is high. For those whose risk is high current treatment targets are to reduce the total cholesterol level to below 4 mmol/l or the LDL-cholesterol to less than 2 mmol/l.

## Assessment of cardiovascular risk

If you have previously had a heart attack, your risk of a further attack is six times higher, because it suggests that blood flow to your heart has already been affected. Under these circumstances, the absolute risk of dying from CVD associated with a cholesterol level of 6.5 mmol/l is over 3 per cent (1 in 33) in middle age.

Most people with angina face a similar risk, and preventing further coronary disease is a high priority. Most angina and heart attack patients will benefit by lowering their cholesterol. The aim is to reduce total cholesterol levels as low as possible, and certainly to below 4 mmol/l.

The risk of CVD is increased by about three times in cigarette smokers and a similar risk is associated with high blood pressure or hypertension. These and other risks multiply together, so that the risk of CVD in a hypertensive patient who smokes is nine times higher than in a person without these risk factors.

Other risk factors, such as high blood cholesterol levels and increasing age, cause this risk to increase steeply, so treatment to reduce cholesterol levels may be suggested even if there is no history of CVD.

## Cardiovascular risk calculators

It is difficult to arrive at an estimate of coronary risk by juggling risk factors in your head, but help is available in the shape of CVD risk calculators. Many of the CVD risk factors identified in the box on page 10 have been included in risk prediction charts, which relate these risk factors to blood cholesterol levels.

Separate charts are available for men and women, reflecting their different cardiovascular risk. The charts (shown on pages 57–9) present the risk of developing CVD over the next 10 years. Patients whose risk falls within the red zone (CVD risk greater than 20 per cent over the next 10 years or 2 per cent per annum) should reduce their risk factors.

Charts are convenient for seeing at a glance whether your risk of CVD is high. Doctors use them, but they can also put the values for the various risk factors into a spreadsheet to calculate the risk more precisely.

Not all risk factors are included. A family history of CVD is a risk factor that is usually left out of risk calculators. Ethnicity is not included and most risk factor calculators are unsuitable for patients with diabetes.

## Who should have blood cholesterol measured?

General screening of the whole adult population for hypercholesterolaemia would prove expensive, not only for the screening programme itself, but also for the extensive facilities needed for effective treatment and follow-up. Mass cholesterol screening is therefore not feasible. In addition, some people could be identified as having 'high' cholesterol levels when their absolute risk of CVD was not particularly great. This would have adverse effects, such as increased anxiety, because such people might perceive themselves as unhealthy.

Blood cholesterol levels are usually measured only when there is an indication to do so, such as signs of:

- hypercholesterolaemia (for example, tendon xanthomas, xanthelasmas or early corneal arcus)
- a personal history of heart disease
- the presence of other CVD risk factors
- a family history of early coronary disease
- a family history of hypercholesterolaemia.

## When should blood cholesterol levels be measured?

Measurements should form part of an overall assessment

# Calculation of cardiovascular disease (CVD) risk

To estimate an individual's absolute 10-year risk of developing CVD, find the table (see pages 58 and 59) for gender, smoking status (smoker/non-smoker) and age.

Then you need to know the person's:

Blood pressure
Total cholesterol (TC)
High-density lipoprotein (HDL) – if unknown assume 1.0 mmol/litre

For example, if you are a 50-year-old man, a non-smoker without diabetes and your:

- Blood pressure = 120/80 mmHg
- Total cholesterol (TC) = 6.2 mmol/litre
- HDL = 1.3 mmol/litre

Then:

Systolic blood pressure (SBP) = 120 mmHg
TC/HDL = 6.2/1.3 = 4.8

From the correct table (see pages 58–9) find the SBP on the vertical axis and the TC/HDL on the horizontal axis and read off the risk value (see example below).

In this case the risk of having a non-fatal or fatal heart attack or stroke is less than 10 per cent over the next 10 years.

## Non-diabetic men

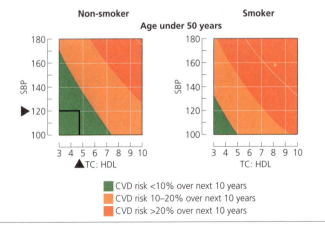

**Non-smoker** | **Smoker**
**Age under 50 years**

CVD risk <10% over next 10 years
CVD risk 10–20% over next 10 years
CVD risk >20% over next 10 years

# Cardiovascular risk prediction charts

See the instructions in the box on page 57 for the method of using these charts to estimate an individual's absolute 10-year risk of developing CVD.

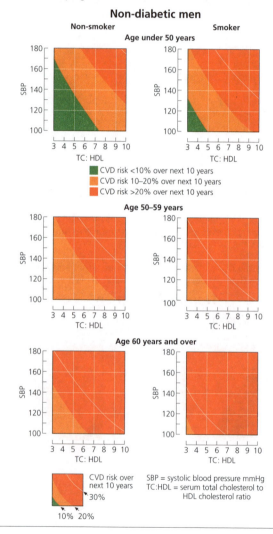

## Non-diabetic men

**Non-smoker**  **Smoker**

### Age under 50 years

- 🟩 CVD risk <10% over next 10 years
- 🟧 CVD risk 10–20% over next 10 years
- 🟥 CVD risk >20% over next 10 years

### Age 50–59 years

### Age 60 years and over

CVD risk over next 10 years
10% 20% 30%

SBP = systolic blood pressure mmHg
TC:HDL = serum total cholesterol to HDL cholesterol ratio

## Cardiovascular risk prediction charts (contd)

See the instructions in the box on page 57 for the method of using these charts to estimate an individual's absolute 10-year risk of developing CVD.

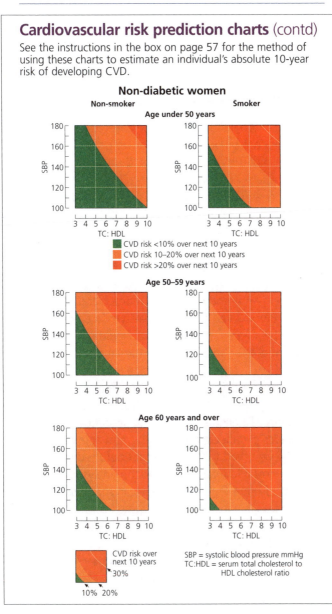

**Non-diabetic women**

SBP = systolic blood pressure mmHg
TC:HDL = serum total cholesterol to
HDL cholesterol ratio

of coronary risk, and blood cholesterol levels are ideally measured in settings where this is available. In addition to CVD risk assessment, advice about diet and lifestyle, and more active treatment measures are needed. This is usually done by your doctor (GP) or by occupational health services at your place of work.

The main points that should be covered in CVD risk assessment are outlined in the box on page 62.

Home cholesterol testing kits and pharmacy testing are not usually accompanied by assessment of other risk factors and on their own may not be helpful. If you suspect that your cholesterol levels are high, it is important to see your GP.

## How is blood cholesterol measured?

Your doctor or nurse will usually take a blood sample from a vein and send it to an accredited laboratory for analysis. Blood levels of total cholesterol are not affected by a recent meal and you would not have to fast overnight for a simple cholesterol measurement.

Your doctor may want to check all your blood lipids at the same time (full blood lipid profile), to assess high-density lipoprotein (HDL)-cholesterol, low-density lipoprotein (LDL)-cholesterol and triglycerides. Triglycerides are affected by a recent meal and you would therefore be asked to fast overnight before the test.

Some portable machines (desk-top analysers) sample the blood from a fingerprick; they can measure lipids and are available in some general practices. If they are used, the results are known during your visit so your coronary risk can be assessed on the spot. Appropriate advice can then be given immediately rather than waiting a few days for information from a laboratory.

## Taking blood for cholesterol measurement

A vein is chosen and the injection site cleaned. A hollow needle attached to a syringe is inserted into the vein and blood drawn out for testing.

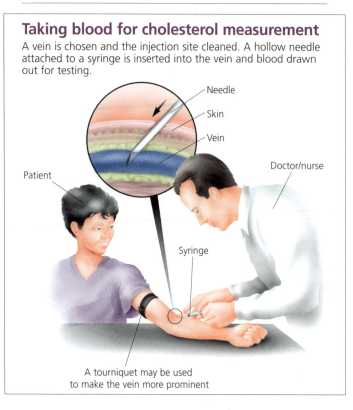

Needle

Skin

Vein

Doctor/nurse

Patient

Syringe

A tourniquet may be used to make the vein more prominent

## When should HDL-cholesterol be measured?

Quite often, your doctor will first get your blood tested for your total cholesterol level – the sum total of all the cholesterol-containing particles in your circulation including LDL- and HDL-cholesterol. If this is satisfactory, no further investigations are required other than to advise a repeat measurement after a few years, just to check whether things have changed.

If your total cholesterol is high, then your HDL-cholesterol is measured as part of a full lipid profile.

## CVD risk assessment

In addition to taking a blood sample to measure your blood cholesterol levels your doctor will need to note the following:

- Gender
- Weight and height
- Personal medical history (diabetes, hypertension, previous heart attack, angina)
- Family history of early CVD or a blood lipid disorder
- Smoking habits
- Alcohol intake
- Diet and exercise patterns
- Blood pressure measurement
- For men, if you are of south Asian origin

This is necessary to find out as much as possible about your lipid abnormality. The average HDL-cholesterol levels in blood are 1.3 mmol/l in men and 1.5 mmol/l in women – this difference is probably the result of differences in the sex hormones.

Your total cholesterol level may be high as a result of a high level of HDL-cholesterol (greater than 2 mmol/l), in which case you are fortunate in that your risk of CVD is not increased. Your CVD risk is increased if your high total cholesterol level is caused by a low HDL-cholesterol concentration (that is, your LDL is high).

Risk calculators for CVD allow for this by expressing the risk from cholesterol as a ratio of total cholesterol to HDL-cholesterol. For example, someone with a total cholesterol level of 8.1 mmol/l and an HDL of 2.1 mmol/l has a total cholesterol:HDL ratio of 8.1/2.1

= 3.8. A total cholesterol:HDL ratio above 6 is associated with increased risk of CVD.

## I don't understand why my cholesterol level has changed

If you have your cholesterol measured regularly, it is quite common to find that the level has changed unexpectedly, without any difference in diet or lifestyle, or changes in therapy. The most probable reason is that, as with all laboratory tests, there is variability in the measurement that cannot be eliminated. Some of this is the result of the measurement process itself (analytical variability) and some is the result of factors inherent in all of us (biological variability).

### Analytical variability

The variation in cholesterol measurement in most accredited laboratories is small, between 1 and 2 per cent. For someone with a cholesterol level of 6.0 mmol/l, such variability would lead to the reading varying from 5.9 to 6.1 mmol/l should no other factor have changed. There is an international programme to ensure that the cholesterol level measured in one accredited laboratory is comparable to one from a second laboratory. Cholesterol levels measured using desk-top analysers are less precise than laboratory measurements and therefore a greater analytical variation results from their use.

### Biological variability

Biological variability causes bigger changes than analytical variability, and cholesterol levels can vary by up to 8 per cent within an individual. A total cholesterol level of 6.0 mmol/l could vary between 5.5

## Biological variability in cholesterol measurement

### Variation in taking the blood sample

For instance, prolonged application of a tourniquet. Blood is taken from a vein after compressing the arm with a tourniquet to make the vein prominent, thus making it easier to insert the needle. If it is difficult to find a vein, the tourniquet is applied for longer than usual and this can lead to apparently higher cholesterol levels because water temporarily filters out of the veins as a result of the pressure.

### Physiological variation

Age and gender can affect it. Blood cholesterol levels increase with age, although the pattern of this increase is different in men and women. For men, the average blood cholesterol level rises until the age of 50 years when it starts falling slightly. Levels are relatively constant in women until they reach menopause when they increase to levels higher than those seen in men.

### Season

Some seasonal changes in cholesterol levels occur, with values around 3 per cent higher in winter than in summer. The reasons for this are not completely clear, but diet seems to be partly responsible.

### Menstrual cycle

Levels vary by as much as 9 per cent during the menstrual cycle, the highest values being seen in the first half of the cycle. This cyclical variation is consistent with the known effects of oestrogens on fat metabolism.

## Biological variability in cholesterol measurement (contd)

### Pregnancy
Cholesterol levels rise quite significantly during pregnancy, again as a result of hormonal changes.

### Lifestyle changes (diet, exercise, alcohol, coffee)
The effect of diet and related lifestyle factors on cholesterol levels is considered on page 75.

### Illness
For example, infection, surgery, heart attack. Any illness can affect cholesterol levels. A heart attack leads to a fall in the blood total cholesterol concentration within 24 hours, the effect lasting several weeks. The reason for this is thought to be stress; this also explains the falls that occur after surgery and major trauma. Even relatively mild illnesses, such as viral infections, can lead to reductions in blood cholesterol levels of up to 15 per cent.

### Malignancy
If a patient has any form of cancer, the blood cholesterol level usually falls. This is probably because tumours grow in an uncontrolled manner and have increased requirements for the building blocks of cells, which include cholesterol.

### Medicines
Some drugs given for other purposes affect cholesterol and other blood fat levels. These are discussed on page 49.

and 6.5 mmol/l as a result of this variability. Biological variability can result from a number of factors. These are outlined in the box on the previous page.

**KEY POINTS**

- Screening everybody for hypercholesterol-aemia is not cost-effective

- Cholesterol should be measured as a part of overall CVD risk assessment

- Cholesterol levels are quite variable within an individual

# Why treat hyper-cholesterolaemia?

Over the last 20 years, the benefits of treating hyper-cholesterolaemia have been demonstrated clearly. Before that, many clinical trials showed inconclusive results because:

- Early treatments were not particularly effective in reducing blood cholesterol levels

- Studies included too few patients to obtain clear results – it is more difficult to get a clear answer from a trial if there have been relatively few clinical events

- Patients who were recruited to studies had a low risk of suffering from cardiovascular disease (CVD).

Since the 1980s, clinical trials have clearly shown the benefits of lowering blood cholesterol levels, particularly if the risk of CVD is high.

## Cholesterol lowering reduces heart attacks

A 1981 study in Norway showed that changing diet to reduce blood lipids and stopping smoking reduced the number of coronary events (mainly heart attacks) by 45 per cent. However, it was difficult in this study to separate the effects of stopping smoking (achieved by 45 per cent of subjects) from those of cholesterol reduction (13 per cent).

Three years later, doctors in America showed that lowering blood cholesterol with the drug cholestyramine reduced the number of heart attacks by 1 per cent in 4,000 middle-aged men, even though the fall in cholesterol was relatively modest at 8.5 per cent.

Similar results were found in Helsinki in 1987 using gemfibrozil, a different type of cholesterol-lowering drug. The blood total cholesterol levels fell 10 per cent whereas the number of coronary events (fatal and non-fatal heart attacks, onset of angina, coronary artery bypass grafts) fell 37 per cent.

These studies suggest that lowering cholesterol reduces coronary events but they did not show a change in death rate. This is important because effective treatment would reduce deaths from CVD. We need to be sure that treatment doesn't increase the rate of other diseases, such as cancer. There are several possible reasons why a change in death rate was not found, the most important being that a relatively small number of individuals were studied for a short period of time using drugs that had a modest cholesterol-lowering effect.

## Cholesterol lowering slows arterial disease

Doctors then studied the effect of cholesterol-lowering treatment on what was happening within arteries. Seven studies published between 1987 and 1994, using different treatments, showed similar results.

Before giving treatment, arterial narrowing caused by plaques was assessed from X-rays.

Follow-up X-rays showed considerably less progression of arterial disease in patients who had received active cholesterol-lowering treatment rather than placebo (dummy tablets). In a small number of patients the size of the abnormalities in the arterial walls actually shrank. Even when the abnormalities did not shrink, it is thought that treatment stabilised the plaques, reducing the risk of thrombosis and complete blockage of the artery.

## Cholesterol lowering improves survival

The first evidence that patients with high total cholesterol levels live longer if cholesterol is reduced came from pooling the results of several clinical trials. This technique is called meta-analysis, and has greater statistical power than individual clinical trials.

Meta-analysis showed that lowering blood cholesterol by 10 per cent in patients with an average cholesterol level of 6 mmol/l produced a 10 per cent reduction in death rates.

Meta-analysis was used as individual trials did not give enough information to support the conclusion because:

- the drugs used produced only modest reductions in cholesterol

- there were too few patients in the individual trials

- the patients were not at particularly high risk from CHD (coronary heart disease) and therefore from the number of cardiac events.

## The results of clinical trials and statins

More recently, powerful cholesterol-lowering drugs, known as statins, have been introduced into general practice and several individual clinical trials have demonstrated clear survival benefits from treatment.

The first trial was the Scandinavian Simvastatin Survival Study (4S), in which 4,444 patients with angina or previous myocardial infarction and blood cholesterol levels of 5.5 to 8.0 millimoles per litre (mmol/l) were given either active treatment with a statin or treatment with a placebo.

There was a reduction of CHD deaths of 42 per cent and overall mortality fell 30 per cent; blood cholesterol fell by almost 30 per cent in those who received simvastatin. Both men and women benefited equally and the relative decrease in CHD was similar in younger and older age groups. These results have been confirmed in other trials in which an alternative statin, pravastatin, has been used.

Trials have also shown that benefits are similar in both smokers and non-smokers, patients with high blood pressure and those with normal blood pressure, patients with and without diabetes and elderly people. Most of these trials have been in patients with existing CHD although one, in Scotland, looked at people without existing CHD. This showed that treatment reduced the incidence of CHD, although the results for survival were not as clear cut, possibly because the study population was at lower risk than in other statin trials.

A further important study using statins has been published recently (the Heart Protection Study). Over 20,000 individuals were included who had arterial disease or diabetes. The death rate was reduced by a third in those who received the drug for up to five years. For patients with diabetes (but without existing vascular disease), there was a reduction of about 25 per cent in the incidence of heart attacks and strokes. The CARDS study also showed that statins prevented heart attacks in patients with diabetes. Atorvastatin was used in this trial.

Statin trials have had a profound effect in emphasising the importance of cholesterol as a risk factor for CHD. There is no doubt that effective reduction of blood cholesterol levels by using these drugs, at least in patients who are at high risk, reduces the incidence of CHD and improves overall survival.

The trials have also shown benefits in preventing ischaemic stroke.

## Does cholesterol lowering do any harm?

This question has received considerable attention in the newspapers and medical press over the years, more so than for related treatments such as the management of hypertension. A related question is whether patients who naturally have a low blood cholesterol level are at increased risk of other diseases, such as cancer, as a result.

### Safety and clinical trials

Initial doubts about the safety of lowering cholesterol related to clinical trials undertaken in the 1980s, which showed that the number of heart attacks was reduced, although there was no overall reduction in the death rate (mortality). Some of these trials even suggested that there were more deaths from suicide and violent deaths in those receiving active intervention compared with the control patients, but the numbers were extremely small and the difference between the two groups was not statistically significant. Despite this, the possibility of a link received some support, particularly as the findings were linked with results of experiments in laboratory animals, which showed that modifying fat intake leads to behavioural changes.

It is obviously important to establish that any disadvantages of a particular treatment are outweighed by the benefits. The issue of suicide and violent deaths has now been looked at in individual studies and by pooling the results of a number of trials using meta-analysis. Individual studies and meta-analysis have not shown any significant increase in the broad category of deaths caused by accidents and suicides, and have failed to show any link between mood and cholesterol lowering. Similarly, no excess deaths from cancer have been shown by meta-analysis.

## Naturally occurring low cholesterol levels

There is a U-shaped relationship between total mortality (death from all causes) and blood cholesterol levels. This graph relates to cholesterol levels without any treatment and could be interpreted as indicating that the overall death rate was higher in people with blood cholesterol levels of 4 mmol/l than in those with a level of 5 mmol/l.

Such an interpretation is incorrect. The reason for the apparently higher mortality in those with low cholesterol levels was early deaths from cancer. Cancer is known to lower cholesterol (see page 65) and therefore the most probable explanation is that the patients already had an undiagnosed malignant disease when the blood sample for cholesterol was taken.

There are other reasons for concluding that low blood cholesterol levels are not harmful and may be beneficial:

- In long-term follow-up (30 years) the higher mortality associated with low cholesterol levels disappears. If low cholesterol levels caused cancer, it would persist.

- Some populations, such as rural Chinese people, have naturally occurring low cholesterol levels without showing excess deaths from malignant disease, suicide or violence.

- Recent clinical trials, including the Heart Protection Study and CARDS, have shown that patients at high risk of CHD benefit from cholesterol reduction with statins even if their cholesterol levels are relatively low (total cholesterol less than 5.0 mmol/l, LDL-cholesterol less than 3.0 mmol/l).

## KEY POINTS

■ Cholesterol reduction prevents heart disease

■ Cholesterol reduction increases length of life

■ Cholesterol reduction does not increase your likelihood of suffering other diseases

# Non-drug treatment of hyper-cholesterolaemia

The reason for treating hypercholesterolaemia is to reduce your risk of cardiovascular disease (CVD), rather than concern that your cholesterol levels should fall within narrow limits. The main treatment to reduce CVD risk is change of diet and lifestyle.

Other conditions, such as high blood pressure, may also need to be treated. If you are at high risk of CVD, you may need to take medication to lower blood cholesterol levels if dietary and lifestyle changes do not improve things sufficiently.

## Lifestyle
Several lifestyle changes reduce the risk of CVD. These include stopping smoking, drinking alcohol in moderation, losing weight and increasing aerobic exercise.

### Cigarette smoking
Cigarette smokers who give up smoking show a rapid

## Changing your lifestyle can reduce your risk of CVD

| Lifestyle change of CVD | Reduction in risk |
|---|---|
| Stopping smoking | 50–70% within 5 years |
| Losing excess weight | 35–55% |
| Exercising for at least 20 minutes, three times a week | 45% |
| Keeping alcohol intakes within healthy limits | 25–45% lower risk than those who drink excessively |
| Not adding salt during cooking or at the table | 15% |

fall in CVD risk (50 per cent in one year), although the level of risk does not approach that in people who have not smoked for many years. Giving up smoking is obviously difficult but can be helped by appropriate support. Nicotine patches or gum has a role, particularly in people who are highly motivated to quit. Quitting smoking doesn't reduce blood cholesterol levels but high cholesterol levels are less likely to cause CHD in people who don't smoke compared with those who do.

## Alcohol consumption

The consequences of excessive alcohol intake are well known. In addition to the effects on social activities, there are clear medical risks, including permanent liver damage, obesity, hypertension and damage to the heart. High alcohol intake is also a risk factor for stroke.

However, there is considerable evidence of benefits from light-to-moderate alcohol consumption, including

## Lifestyle changes

You can do a lot to help your long-term health by making simple lifestyle changes: maintain the correct weight for your height, stop smoking, drink alcohol in moderation, eat plenty of fruit and vegetables, and take regular exercise.

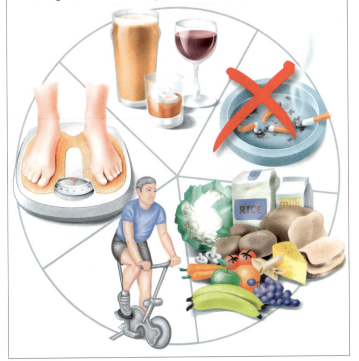

lower mortality, as a result of a reduced risk of CVD, particularly coronary heart disease (CHD). Benefits for women are found at lower levels of alcohol intake than for men and are most pronounced in postmenopausal women. This is not surprising because the incidence of CVD increases after the menopause, and therefore the absolute risk is higher in this age group than in younger women.

## Alcohol and mortality

Graph showing the approximate relationship between alcohol consumption and mortality for men and women.

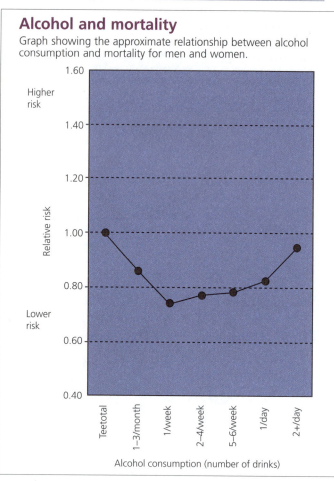

Some reports have suggested that the beneficial effects of drinking alcohol are related to the type of drink – for example, that drinking red wine gave more benefit than other alcoholic drinks because of the anti-oxidants that it contained. Recent studies have shown that the benefits occur in those who drink wine, beer or spirits in moderation, and are largely independent of type.

The main benefit therefore appears to result from alcohol itself, rather than from other components. Drinking moderate amounts of alcohol affects your cholesterol metabolism, raising your HDL-cholesterol levels. It is possible that alcohol protects through other mechanisms, such as preventing blood clotting and improving the state of your artery walls.

What is moderate alcohol consumption? The usual recommendations are that men should drink no more than 21 units of alcohol spread over the course of a week, and women no more than 14 units. One glass of wine, a pub single measure of spirits or half a pint of beer contains one unit.

## Weight

The healthy weight range for people of different heights is worked out clinically using the body mass

### What is a unit of alcohol?

A one-litre bottle of spirits – brandy, whisky or gin – contains about 40 units of alcohol

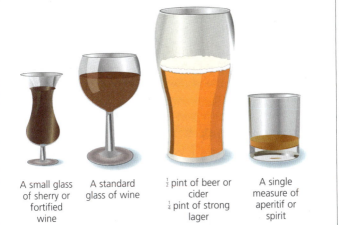

A small glass of sherry or fortified wine

A standard glass of wine

½ pint of beer or cider
¼ pint of strong lager

A single measure of aperitif or spirit

index (BMI) formula:

BMI = Weight (kg)/[Height × Height (m²)]

If this calculation gives a result between 18.5 and 24.9, you are in the healthy weight range for your height – this means that your weight is not increasing your risk of premature death, especially from CVD.

If your BMI is less than 18.5, you are underweight and if it is 25 to 29.9 you are overweight. If it is 30 or above, you are classed as obese, and your risk of dying prematurely is double that of someone in the healthy weight range. These BMI calculations are widely used for all adults, although the ranges are slightly smaller for women.

## Exercise

People who are physically active are less likely to develop CVD than those who are not. The good news is that the greatest benefit comes from being moderately active – the extra gain from vigorous or prolonged exercise regimes is small. Types of exercise that are beneficial include brisk walking, dancing or reasonably heavy gardening. The protective effect is lost if you stop exercising.

The reasons for the beneficial effects of exercise are not completely clear but probably include weight reduction, lower blood pressure and increasing your blood levels of HDL-cholesterol.

## Dietary changes

The cholesterol in our circulation comes from two sources. Small amounts are obtained pre-formed from certain foods such as egg yolk and meat products, but most is made in your liver from saturated fats (animal and dairy fat), so a diet high in saturated fats raises

# What should you weigh?

- The body mass index (BMI) is a useful measure of healthy weight
- Find out your height in metres and weight in kilograms
- Calculate your BMI like this:

$$BMI = \frac{\text{Your weight (kg)}}{[\text{Your height (metres)} \times \text{Your height (metres)}]}$$

$$\text{e.g. } 24.8 = \frac{70}{[1.68 \times 1.68]}$$

- You are recommended to try to maintain a BMI in the range 18.5–24.9
- The chart below is an easier way of estimating your BMI. Read off your height and your weight. The point where the lines cross in the chart indicates your BMI

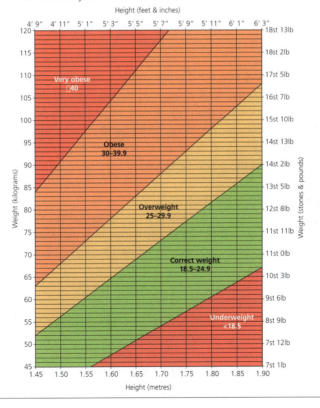

blood cholesterol levels.

Changing your diet is therefore essential for reducing blood cholesterol levels, whatever their cause. There are two main dietary approaches:

- generally reducing the amount of fat that you eat
- using or avoiding specific foods or additives.

## General dietary changes

You may need to change your diet to reduce your saturated fat intake but you may also need to adjust it so that you lose weight. Fat is the richest source of calories in your diet. On average in the UK, over 40 per cent of the calories in our food comes from fat.

Healthy eating guidelines for the general population recommend that fat should contribute less than 35 per cent of calories. This is reduced to less than 30 per cent for those at high risk from CVD, including people with hypercholesterolaemia. The general principles of the dietary approach to reducing cholesterol are outlined in the box on page 85.

### Low-cholesterol diet

People often talk about a 'low-cholesterol diet'. What they really mean is a cholesterol-lowering diet. 'Low-cholesterol diet' implies that reducing cholesterol intake is the objective of the diet.

### Where does cholesterol come from?

Although the amount of cholesterol in your diet is important, it is probably less so than the amount of saturated fat that you eat, because most cholesterol in your body is made in the liver from dietary saturated fats.

Cholesterol is also absorbed rather poorly from the gut, with over half remaining behind. The main objective of changing your diet is to reduce your saturated fat intake. However, saturated fat and cholesterol tend to occur in high amounts in the same foods, so by avoiding fat you are probably also lowering your intake of cholesterol.

## The atherogenic index

The fat content of food is expressed here as an atherogenic index. This method of expressing fat content gives high values for foods rich in saturated fat (increases risk of CVD). The greater the proportion of unsaturated fat the lower the value (reduces risk of CVD).

| Food | Atherogenic index |
| --- | --- |
| Cheese, full fat | 2.0 |
| Butter | 2.0 |
| Lamb, roast | 1.0 |
| Lamb, lean chop | 1.0 |
| Beef, roast lean topside | 0.7 |
| Beef, uncooked mince | 0.7 |
| Bacon, streaky fried | 0.7 |
| Pork, roast lean | 0.6 |
| Pork sausages, grilled | 0.6 |
| Chicken, roast | 0.5 |
| Polyunsaturated margarine | 0.4 |
| Mackerel, uncooked | 0.3 |
| Olive oil | 0.1 |
| Sunflower oil | 0.1 |

As the intake of saturated fats (animal and dairy fat) is more important than that of cholesterol, foods rich in cholesterol with a modest amount of saturated fats are allowed in moderation, including eggs and shellfish. It is OK to eat two eggs and one portion of shellfish per week.

### Fibre

Dietary fibre, which consists of carbohydrates resistant to our digestive enzymes, is found in fruit, vegetables and wholegrain cereals. Fibre intake is associated with a protective effect against CVD.

One study in America followed 75,521 female nurses for 10 years, having established their intake of fibre before and during the period of investigation. The relationship of fibre intake to CVD was studied after adjusting the results for other factors that could affect the incidence of CVD, such as smoking, age, weight, alcohol intake, HRT usage, vitamin intake and exercise.

The nurses with the highest intake of wholegrains had the lowest incidence of CVD. These results have been confirmed in other studies. This protective effect is related to the effects of dietary fibre on the absorption of fats in the gut, resulting in lower LDL-cholesterol levels. Three grams of fibre per day in the form of oats can lower cholesterol by around 0.15 mmol/litre.

### Fish and fish oils

There is strong evidence that people who eat fish are at lower risk of developing CVD than those who do not. This was first noticed in Greenland Eskimos who eat a diet with a very high fat content from seal, whale and fish, yet have a low incidence of CVD.

This is now known to be the result of a type of polyunsaturated fat, known as omega-3 fatty acids, of which two are found in fish oils: eicosapentaenoic acid (EPA) and docosahexaenoic acid (DHA). EPA and DHA are found in large amounts in fish and sea mammals, but are almost absent from land animals and plants because they are not produced by marine animals themselves, but by microscopic plankton that are at the base of the marine food chain.

## General principles of a cholesterol-lowering diet (high fibre)

- Lose weight if your weight is increased
- Remember that alcohol has lots of calories
- Eat plenty of fresh fruit and vegetables – at least five portions per day
- Limit red meat, eat more chicken and fish
- Use margarine made from stanol esters (see page 86), olive oil or one high in polyunsaturates
- Use skimmed or semi-skimmed milk
- Avoid lard; use olive oil or an oil that is high in polyunsaturated fats for cooking, for example, corn, sunflower or soya oil
- Include wholemeal bread, cereals, pasta and rice in your diet
- Cut down on all animal fats – they are rich in saturated fatty acids
- Animal and vegetable proteins have little effect on cholesterol levels
- You are allowed treats, including eggs, occasionally!

Fish oils with high amounts of EPA and DHA, but with fat-soluble vitamins removed (which could be toxic in high doses), are available from health food shops. Untreated cod liver oil contains fat-soluble vitamins.

It is unlikely that the major benefits of fish and fish oil result from their effect on blood lipids – they have little effect on cholesterol, although they do reduce blood triglyceride levels. However, they have a number of anti-clotting effects and help to prevent abnormal heart rhythms developing. Fish oils also improve the health of the walls of arteries and lessen atherosclerotic plaque formation.

It used to be thought that fish and fish oils should not be increased in patients with diabetes because they could make diabetes more difficult to control. This is now thought not to be the case, provided that the total number of calories is not increased.

## Specific foods and additives

Foods obviously contain essential nutrients, but they also contain substances that are not nutrients but have properties that are potentially useful. Less attention has been paid to the effect of individual foods on blood cholesterol and the risk of CVD than to fat intake.

The notion that natural remedies, such as specific foods or drinks, can lessen CVD risk is extremely attractive. However, it is equally possible that a relatively high intake of specific foodstuffs could be harmful – remember the effect of saturated fatty acids. Specific foodstuffs and natural remedies should be assessed as rigorously as drugs.

### Margarine containing stanol esters

Cholesterol is a sterol and similar compounds with

slightly different structures are found in plants. As they have a similar structure, plant sterols, particularly a group called stanol esters, can interfere with the absorption of cholesterol.

Stanol esters such as sitostanol have been used in a chemically modified form in mayonnaises or margarines, such as Benecol and Flora pro.activ. Several clinical studies have shown that this type of margarine lowers blood cholesterol levels. For example, a study in people with mildly elevated blood cholesterol levels showed that it lowers the total cholesterol level by around 10 per cent when used in relatively small amounts of three grams a day. Very little stanol is absorbed into the body and the major effect appears to be by reducing cholesterol absorption from the gut. Stanol-containing yoghurts and drinks are now available.

## Antioxidants

These are of interest because chemical change in LDL by a process called oxidation increases the uptake of LDL particles by scavenger cells in arterial walls, forming the basis of atherosclerotic lesions. Antioxidants prevent these changes in LDL, at least in the laboratory.

Dietary antioxidants include vitamins A, C and E, and polyphenols. Garlic also has antioxidant properties (see below). There are two points about dietary antioxidants to consider:

- whether the amount in the natural diet affects CVD risk
- whether the addition of antioxidant dietary supplements has any benefit.

Observational studies relating vitamin E or vitamin C intake to CVD are contradictory, with some suggesting benefit and some not. Studies in which high doses of vitamin E or beta-carotene (one form of vitamin A) were added to the diet have been disappointing.

In addition to studying statins (see page 70), the Heart Protection Study also looked at whether vitamin E supplements prevented heart attacks. There was no benefit at all from the extra vitamin.

Polyphenols are a type of antioxidant found in drinks such as black or green tea and red wine. The beneficial effects of red wine seem to be shared with other alcoholic drinks that do not have high contents of polyphenols. So far there is not enough known about the effects of polyphenols but studies are being made of plant extracts given to animals and the early results are encouraging, although it is too early to recommend them for human use.

Some metals, particularly copper, manganese, zinc and selenium, are involved in antioxidant processes within the body. Only small amounts of these are required in a healthy diet – this is why they are called trace metals. There is no clinical evidence that dietary supplements of these trace metals are of any value in preventing CVD.

Overall, the case for dietary antioxidants is unproven.

## Garlic

Some people believe that garlic may be useful in reducing the risk of CVD through an effect on cardiovascular risk factors. There are several reasons for this, one of which is that garlic consumption is high in areas where the risk of CVD is low. This doesn't prove that garlic is protective because other factors are also different in these areas, such as a low intake of saturated fat in the diet.

Garlic has several properties that may be beneficial. These include reducing the tendency for blood to clot, reducing blood pressure and lowering levels of fats in blood. In addition, garlic has antioxidant activity.

Some articles in the medical literature suggest that a powder prepared from garlic lowers cholesterol, although two recent high-quality studies do not confirm this. These are important because they include more participants than previous investigations. If trials are added together, the overall effect is small, a reduction of 0.1 mmol.

We do not yet have enough information on the other possible effects of garlic, such as on blood clotting or through antioxidant activity, to judge its possible benefit. In addition, garlic has not been investigated to see whether it reduces the incidence of heart attacks. The present situation is therefore that there is no proven benefit from eating garlic to prevent CVD.

## Avocados

Avocados are rich in monounsaturated fatty acids and avocado oil has a composition closely resembling that of olive oil. They contain no cholesterol. Avocados are therefore thought to be beneficial in a diet to prevent CVD.

## Coffee

There has been considerable controversy about the effect of coffee on blood lipids and, in particular, cholesterol levels. The effect appears to relate to the type of coffee beans and the method used to prepare the drink.

Blood cholesterol levels are about 15 per cent higher in men who drink 10 or more cups of coffee a day, made by boiling beans, compared with non-coffee drinkers. The substances responsible are cafestol and kahweol, which are from a group of chemicals called diterpenes.

The types of brew that have a cholesterol-raising effect are Turkish coffee, Scandinavian boiled coffee and cafetière coffee. The effect is not seen in those who drink instant or filtered coffee. It seems sensible to avoid drinking lots of boiled coffee, although it is unlikely that an occasional cup of cafetière coffee will do much harm.

## Herbal remedies

There is a great deal of interest in herbal remedies such as hawthorn extracts, red yeast rice, guggul, fenugreek and artichoke. Some of these, particularly fenugreek seeds, do appear to have cholesterol-lowering properties, although there is no evidence of benefit, in terms of a reduced incidence of CVD.

## Vitamins

Vitamins A and E have been discussed above. There is some evidence that patients with low blood levels of folate (a type of vitamin B) have a greater risk of CVD than those with higher levels. Rich dietary sources of folate are breakfast cereals, fruit, green vegetables and beans (legumes). It is difficult to know, however, whether folate has an independent effect on blood cholesterol levels or whether it is a marker for some other component of diet, such as fibre.

There is a further factor that may be important in relation to folate. High blood levels of the amino acid, homocysteine, appear to damage artery walls, increasing the risk of arterial disease. Folate reduces homocysteine in blood and high folate concentrations could protect against arterial disease by this mechanism. However, for the present, this is speculation.

## Grapefruit

Grapefruit is unique among fruit and vegetables in increasing blood levels of many drugs, which increases their potency. This effect occurs because grapefruit (and grapefruit juice) contains a substance or substances that slow the removal of drugs from the body by the liver.

In addition, there is the possibility of interactions with prescribed drugs and side effects have been described, including abdominal upsets and low blood potassium levels.

The best advice is to avoid grapefruit and grapefruit juice if you are taking any of the drugs affected, which includes statins (see box). Countries that include grapefruit warnings on labels include New Zealand, Australia and the Netherlands. It is possible that there are more grapefruit–drug interactions that are not yet recognised.

---

**Some drugs that carry a grapefruit interaction warning**

- Sedatives (alprazolam, midazolam)
- Cholesterol-lowering drugs (statins)
- Drugs used in the treatment of angina and hypertension (amlodipine, nifedipine, verapamil)
- Oral contraceptive components (ethinyloestradiol)
- Antidepressants (clomipramine)
- Others (ciclosporin, tacrolimus)

### Specific diets

Specific diets, such as the Atkins and GI diets, often receive considerable publicity. The Atkins diet is low in carbohydrate and high in fat and, on this basis, cannot be recommended.

The abbreviation GI stands for glycaemic (or sugar) index and is a measure of the amount that the blood sugar level rises after eating that food. Bread and sugar have an index of 100, whereas the value for baked beans is 69 and for an apple 52. There is no evidence that low GI diets have any effect on blood cholesterol levels.

### Professional dietary advice

Should you see a dietitian? Dietitians are very knowledgeable about the right and wrong sorts of food to eat. They are better than doctors at lowering blood cholesterol through dietary advice although similar reductions can be achieved using self-help resources, if the basic principles are understood.

## KEY POINTS

- The main treatment to reduce CHD risk is change of diet and lifestyle

- Diet is the cornerstone of treatment to reduce blood cholesterol levels

- Stop smoking

- Drink alcohol in moderation

- Maintain a healthy body weight

- Take regular exercise

- Reduce the amount of animal and dairy fat that you eat

# Drug treatment of hypercholesterol-aemia

Drug treatment for hypercholesterolaemia is considered when lifestyle and dietary changes have been tried but failed to reduce the absolute risk of CVD (cardiovascular disease) sufficiently. The decision to start treatment should be made after a discussion between you and your doctor, during which benefits and possible risks can be aired. Treatment should be considered where the risk is more than 20 per cent over a 10-year period or above 2 per cent per year. In general, you will fall into this category if you have CVD, diabetes or more than one risk factor.

Two main groups of drugs lower blood lipid levels: statins and fibrates. Other drugs are used more rarely, including resins and nicotinic acid (see box on page 99).

## Statins
Statins are good at lowering blood cholesterol levels, often by 40 per cent or more, but have less activity against triglycerides (see page 107). They work by

## How statins work

Statins are very effective at reducing blood cholesterol levels. They work by reducing the amount of cholesterol that cells make internally, forcing cells to absorb more cholesterol from outside.

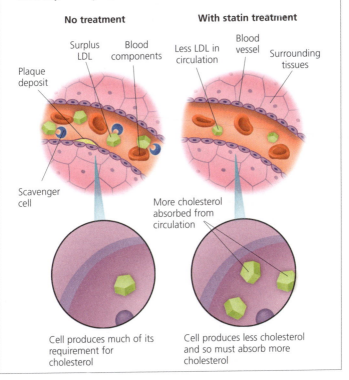

**No treatment**

Plaque deposit

Surplus LDL

Blood components

Scavenger cell

**With statin treatment**

Less LDL in circulation

Blood vessel

Surrounding tissues

More cholesterol absorbed from circulation

Cell produces much of its requirement for cholesterol

Cell produces less cholesterol and so must absorb more cholesterol

reducing the amount of cholesterol made inside body cells, especially in the liver, which in turn increases their production of LDL receptors because they have to obtain a greater proportion of their cholesterol needs from the circulation. As a result, more LDL particles are taken up through cell walls. This removes more cholesterol-rich LDL particles from the blood, and reduces blood cholesterol levels.

Statins are not very good at reducing blood triglyceride levels or increasing HDL-cholesterol concentrations. It is possible that statins have other beneficial effects, including improving the state of arterial walls.

Statins are normally taken as tablets or capsules once a day in the evening, because our bodies make slightly more cholesterol at night than during the day. Treatment is adjusted to bring your total cholesterol level to below 4 millimoles per litre (mmol/l) and the LDL-cholesterol to below 2 mmol/l.

There are some differences between the statins that may lead your doctor to choose a particular drug. Those prescribed most frequently are simvastatin and atorvastatin.

## Side effects of statins

Statins are generally well tolerated, producing few side effects. A small number of people develop muscle aches and pains, as a result of inflammation. Very occasionally this reaction may be severe, in which case treatment should be changed. Frequently, use of an alternative statin will solve this problem.

A mild type of liver inflammation (hepatitis) may also occur when treatment is started, but it usually clears by itself. Occasionally, more severe hepatitis can occur which requires a change in treatment.

Some patients suffer from indigestion. A very rare side effect in men is erectile dysfunction. Some people suffer disturbance of their sleep pattern which may be resolved by taking their tablets in the morning instead of the evening.

Statins should not be taken during pregnancy or breast-feeding. Avoid grapefruits and grapefruit juice if you are taking statins.

## Statins over the counter

Simvastatin is now available over the counter at pharmacies. This is not suitable if you have heart disease, diabetes, familial hypercholesterolaemia or other risk factors because you need to be under the care of your GP who will ensure that treatment is appropriate for your level of risk.

Over-the-counter statins are appropriate if you have a moderate risk, for example, a single risk factor. The dose (10 mg) is lower than is usually given by a doctor and you need to bear in mind that simvastatin is not a magic bullet. It doesn't replace a sensible diet and lifestyle. However, the availability does offer an option to those of some, but not high, risk of CVD.

# Ezetimibe

A new class of cholesterol-lowering drugs, absorption inhibitors, has been introduced recently. The first drug in this class, ezetimibe, lowers LDL-cholesterol levels by 10 to 20 per cent as a single therapy, but it can also be prescribed with statins. The cholesterol-lowering effect of ezetimibe adds to that of statins, with reductions in LDL-cholesterol of 60 per cent being found with the combination.

Ezetimibe appears to be safe from published studies. It is unclear how much of its cholesterol-lowering effect is the result of a reduction in the absorption of dietary cholesterol and how much results from blockage of recycling of cholesterol between the liver and the gut.

It is recommended as a single treatment when patients can't tolerate statins, or combined with statins when the cholesterol level needs to be lowered further.

## Fibrates

Fibrates lower cholesterol levels less than statins, but are more effective in reducing blood triglyceride concentrations. They work by reducing the rate at which lipoprotein-rich particles found in the blood are produced, and by increasing the rate at which they are removed. They also increase circulating levels of 'good' HDL-cholesterol.

Fibrates are taken as tablets or capsules. For people with very severe hyperlipidaemia they are occasionally given with statins, although this does increase the risk of side effects. They can reduce LDL-cholesterol levels by up to 18 per cent.

## Side effects of fibrates

Fibrates are usually well tolerated although they can sometimes cause indigestion or nausea. Skin rashes and impotence are rare side effects. The risk of inflamed muscles with statin treatment is a little greater if fibrates are also given.

## Other drugs

Statins and fibrates are the main drugs used to treat hypercholesterolaemia although others are used occasionally.

Resins are taken as powder or granules dissolved in water. They stay in the gut, binding bile acids so that they can no longer be reabsorbed. As a result of this, more cholesterol is converted to bile acids in the liver, so draining cholesterol from the body.

Before statins became available, the resins were the main drug treatment for hypercholesterolaemia and high doses were used. In general, they were tolerated poorly causing digestive upsets such as indigestion and

## Drugs used to treat hypercholesterolaemia in the UK

| Drug group | Generic names | Trade names |
|---|---|---|
| Statins | simvastatin<br>atorvastatin<br>pravastatin<br>fluvastatin<br>rosuvastatin | Zocor<br>Lipitor<br>Lipostat<br>Lescol<br>Crestor |
| Fibrates | bezafibrate<br>ciprofibrate<br>gemfibrozil<br>fenofibrate | Bezalip<br>Modalim<br>Lopid<br>Lipantil |
| Resins | cholestyramine<br>colestipol | Questran<br>Colestid |
| Cholesterol absorption inhibitors | ezetimibe | Ezetrol |
| Others | nicotinic acid<br>acipimox | Nicotinic Acid Tablets<br>Olbetam<br>Niaspan |

diarrhoea. Despite this, they still have a place in treating very severe hypercholesterolaemia, most commonly as an additional treatment to statins in low doses. They complement the cholesterol-lowering effect of statins and there are fewer side effects with the lower doses. However, side effects still occur and the use of resins in this role has now been largely superseded by the use of ezetimibe (cholesterol absorption inhibitor).

## Nicotinic acid

Nicotinic acid is less widely used. This is a type of vitamin B that is required in small amounts. It reduces both cholesterol and triglyceride levels if used in extremely high doses and also raises HDL-cholesterol levels. It is not used much in this country because it can produce frequent, unpleasant side effects, particularly flushing affecting the face, and indigestion. A slow release form, acipimox, is available as is an extended release form, Niaspan. These produce fewer side effects, although they still occur.

## New drug treatments

Interest is developing in drugs that raise HDL-cholesterol levels and a clinical trial of one such agent, torcetrapib, has been reported recently. It was used with a statin and raised HDL-cholesterol levels in people in whom they were low. However, treatment with torcetrapib did not improve life expectancy; indeed more patients died early when receiving the drug. This shows the importance of treating risk rather than just trying to improve blood lipid levels.

# Hormone replacement therapy

Over 40 million women worldwide use hormone replacement therapy (HRT), primarily as treatment for menopausal symptoms. There are other health benefits from HRT, including the prevention of osteoporosis, and there is considerable interest in whether HRT reduces the incidence of CVD.

The incidence of CVD in women rises after the menopause and it is therefore plausible that HRT could prevent CVD. In addition, oestrogens reduce LDL-cholesterol and increase HDL-cholesterol. Some studies, comparing the incidence of CVD in women taking HRT with that in women on no treatment, suggested that it was lower in those receiving HRT. These studies were not designed to investigate the effects of HRT on CVD incidence, however, and the result was a chance finding.

A clinical trial was set up specifically to investigate whether HRT reduces CVD incidence in 2,700 women who already had heart disease and were therefore at extremely high risk of recurrence. Participants were assigned to receive either HRT or inactive placebo and followed for five years. There was no difference in outcome between the two groups.

So the specific trial did not support the previous chance findings of lower rates of CVD in women taking HRT. This is important because this type of randomised trial, in which patients receive either active treatment or a dummy tablet, is viewed as the gold standard for judging the benefits of drug treatment.

The position at present with regard to a possible role for HRT in preventing CVD is that it is not proven.

## KEY POINTS

- The main purpose in treating hypercholesterolaemia is to reduce CVD risk

- Statins are the most powerful cholesterol-lowering drugs

- Addressing other CVD risk factors is also important

- A recent trial suggests that HRT may not protect against CVD as was previously thought

# Special cases

## Familial hypercholesterolaemia: implications for the family

The chances of passing on the gene responsible for familial hypercholesterolaemia to a child are one in two. As the risk of developing early coronary heart disease (CHD) in familial hypercholesterolaemia is very high, it is sensible to identify affected children by measuring their blood cholesterol level. If the total cholesterol level is greater than 6.8 millimoles per litre (mmol/l) in childhood, there is a high probability of familial hypercholesterolaemia.

The abnormality can usually be detected from infancy onwards, although the age at which testing is undertaken depends on the wishes of the parents and the likely age of onset of CHD in the family. Testing may be delayed if the whole family is receiving an appropriate diet but ought to be undertaken by 10 years of age for two reasons. First, compliance with diet is better when introduced early and, second, some children may benefit from drug treatment.

Other conditions with raised blood cholesterol levels, such as polygenic hypercholesterolaemia, are not apparent in early childhood and little is gained by testing blood levels until after puberty.

## Treatment of children with familial hypercholesterolaemia

As with adults, diet forms the basis of treatment, although it is important that any dietary approach supports normal growth and development. In practice, it is important to ensure that the intake of energy is sufficient but not excessive, as even moderate obesity may exacerbate hypercholesterolaemia. The intake of saturated fats should be as low as possible through the measures shown in the box on page 85. Advice should also be given on avoiding other risk factors for CHD, such as smoking.

Drug treatment is sometimes recommended in children, particularly when there is a history of early onset CHD in the family. Resins are usually recommended, because they are not absorbed and thus have less potential for side effects. However, children may not like taking them and they can cause indigestion and altered bowel function. Statins are usually avoided because little is known about their effects on growth and development. There are some reports on the use of statins that suggest that they are effective and well tolerated, and don't interfere with growth and development. However, these were for short periods of time and included relatively few patients.

# Cholesterol-lowering drugs in pregnancy

There is no evidence that cholesterol-lowering drugs affect the development of an unborn baby. However, it is not worth taking any risks and it is usually recommended that women of child-bearing age should use an effective method of contraception if taking cholesterol-lowering drugs.

If a woman with familial hypercholesterolaemia wishes to start a family, she should stop any drug treatment until after the baby is born. This ensures that there is no risk to the baby, and the mother's risk of CHD is unlikely to increase significantly as a result of the period without drugs. Total cholesterol and LDL-cholesterol levels increase in the final stages of pregnancy and during breast-feeding, although they return to previous levels after weaning. It is not known whether these relatively short-term changes increase CHD risk.

## Oral contraception

Early combined oral contraceptives (including oestrogens and progestogens) increase blood levels of cholesterol and triglycerides. However, newer preparations use lower doses and different types of hormones, which do not affect cholesterol levels. Some types produce small increases in triglycerides.

## Rare types of hypercholesterolaemia

The common primary forms of hypercholesterolaemia are familial hypercholesterolaemia, polygenic hyper-cholesterolaemia and familial combined hyperlipidaemia. Rarer forms also occur, some of which relate to abnormalities of the protein components of lipoprotein particles. In general, these rarer abnormalities are associated with an increased risk of early CHD, similar to that seen in familial hypercholesterolaemia. They are picked up by measuring blood cholesterol levels using the principles outlined on pages 56–63.

## Severe hypertriglyceridaemia

Most of this book has been concerned with hyper-cholesterolaemia and hypertriglyceridaemia has been mentioned where it is associated with what is primarily a problem with cholesterol. Blood triglyceride levels are usually less than 2 mmol/l, although higher levels commonly occur after a meal, particularly if the meal contains a lot of fat. These levels rarely exceed 5 mmol/l.

More severe hypertriglyceridaemia can occur, with levels over 20 mmol/l. These can be the result of some other problem, such as diabetes mellitus, particularly when this is poorly controlled, type 1 (early onset) diabetes. Blood triglyceride levels usually improve when the diabetes is well controlled. Alcohol abuse can also cause extremely high blood triglyceride levels, the treatment being severely curtailing alcohol intake.

Very rarely, severe hypertriglyceridaemia can be the result of a defective gene, the one that controls the removal of dietary fat from the bloodstream and its storage in adipose tissue. As triglycerides are not removed from the blood in this condition, the blood serum contains more fat and looks very milky. This is sometimes picked up when a blood sample is taken for another test. The condition is treated by very-low-fat diets.

### Risks of severe hypertriglyceridaemia

Severe hypertriglyceridaemia (blood triglyceride levels greater than 10 mmol/l) increases the risk of pancreatitis. The pancreas is a large gland at the back of the abdomen that produces enzymes to digest food and also hormones such as insulin. The pancreas may become damaged and the enzymes that are normally secreted into the gut are activated within the gland, leading to its partial destruction, pancreatitis. This is a serious condition that is extremely painful.

## Raised blood triglycerides as a risk factor for cardiovascular disease

Blood triglyceride levels are usually less than 2 mmol/l and are considered to be raised if they exceed 2.3 mmol/l in a sample taken after fasting for at least 12 hours. The risks of severe hypertriglyceridaemia (levels greater than 10 mmol/l) are considered above.

Severe hypertriglyceridaemia is uncommon. There has been uncertainty about whether more modestly raised triglyceride levels, seen more commonly, are a risk factor for CVD. In some studies, raised blood triglyceride levels are associated with CVD, although it is difficult to be sure whether this relationship is independent of other risk factors. This is because blood total cholesterol levels are often raised when triglyceride concentrations are increased and HDL-cholesterol levels are usually low under these circumstances.

Using the statistical technique of meta-analysis (combining the results of many studies) it appears that triglycerides are an independent risk factor, particularly in women and patients with diabetes, after adjusting for the risk from low HDL levels.

The most appropriate advice is that blood triglyceride levels should be less than 2 mmol/l. Weight reduction and avoiding fatty foods may be necessary to achieve this, and sometimes treatment with drugs will be appropriate, should dietary measures not be sufficient.

## KEY POINTS

■ Children with familial hypercholesterol-aemia should follow a low-fat diet and avoid other CVD risk factors

■ Severe hypertriglyceridaemia predisposes to pancreatitis

■ Raised triglyceride levels are a risk for CVD in women and people with diabetes

# Useful addresses

We have included the following organisations because, on preliminary investigation, they may be of use to the reader. However, we do not have first-hand experience of each organisation and so cannot guarantee the organisation's integrity. The reader must therefore exercise his or her own discretion and judgement when making further enquiries.

## Benefits Enquiry Line

Tel: 0800 882200
Minicom: 0800 243355
Website: www.dwp.gov.uk
N. Ireland: 0800 220674

Government agency giving information and advice on sickness and disability benefits for people with disabilities and their carers.

## Blood Pressure Association

60 Cranmer Terrace
London SW17 0QS
Tel: 020 8772 4994

Information line: 0845 241 0989 (Mon–Fri 11am–3pm)
Website: www.bpassoc.org.uk

For the best internet advice. Regularly issues press statements when any new information becomes available and has advice leaflets on all aspects of hypertension (for example, pregnancy, renal disease, heart disease). Raises public awareness about, and offers information and support to, people affected by high blood pressure and health-care professionals. Has a wide selection of literature and membership scheme. Please send large A4 SAE and two first-class stamps for information.

### British Heart Foundation

Greater London House, 180 Hampstead Road
London NW1 7AW
Tel: 020 7554 0000
Helpline: 0300 330 3311 (Mon–Fri 9am–6pm)
Website: www.bhf.org.uk

Funds research, promotes education and raises money to buy equipment to treat heart disease. Information and support available for people with heart conditions. Via Heartstart UK arranges training in emergency life-saving techniques for lay people.

### British Nutrition Foundation

High Holborn House, 52–54 High Holborn
London WC1V 6RQ
Tel: 020 7404 6504
Website: www.nutrition.org.uk

Professional association which determines the scientific consensus in nutrition and communicates this through its free publications. An s.a.e. requested for information as no telephone advice is available.

## Chest, Heart & Stroke Scotland

Head office: 65 North Castle Street
Edinburgh EH2 3LT
Tel: 0131 225 5963
Advice line: 0845 077 6000
Website: www.chss.org.uk

Funds research, provides care and support throughout Scotland, and has an advice line to professional advice from trained nurse. Booklets, factsheets, DVDs and videos available free to patients and carers.

## Chest, Heart & Stroke, Northern Ireland

21 Dublin Road
Belfast BT2 7HB
Tel: 028 9032 0184
Helpline: 0845 769 7299
Website: www.nichsa.com

Aims to promote the prevention of, and alleviate the suffering resulting from, chest, heart and stroke illnesses in Northern Ireland through advice and information.

## Clinical Knowledge Summaries

Sowerby Centre for Health Informatics at Newcastle (SCHIN Ltd)
Bede House, All Saints Business Centre
Newcastle upon Tyne NE1 2ES

Tel: 0191 243 6100
Website: www.cks.library.nhs.uk

A website mainly for GPs giving information for patients listed by disease plus named self-help organisations.

## DVLA

Driver and Vehicle Licensing Agency
Swansea SA6 7JL
Tel: 0870 600 0301
Website: www.dvla.gov.uk

Provides information about medical conditions, driving licences, learning to drive, entitlement to drive, endorsements/disqualifications, driving abroad and what to do when you have changed your address and/or name.

## HEART UK

7 North Road
Maidenhead, Berks SL6 1PE
Tel: 0845 450 5988
Website: www.heartuk.org.uk

Offers information, advice and support to people with coronary heart disease and especially those at high risk of familial hypercholesterolaemia. Members receive bi-monthly magazine. Merged with British Hyperlipidaemia Association in June 2002.

## Institute for Complementary and Natural Medicine

Can-Mezzanine, 32–36 Loman Street
London SE1 0EH

Tel: 020 7922 7980
Website: www.i-c-m.org.uk

Umbrella group for complementary medicine organisations. Offers informed, safe choice to public.

## National Institute for Health and Clinical Excellence (NICE)
MidCity Place, 71 High Holborn
London WC1V 6NA
Tel: 0845 003 7780
Website: www.nice.org.uk

Provides national guidance on the promotion of good health and treatment of ill-health. Patient information leaflets are available for each piece of guidance issued.

## NHS Direct
Tel: 0845 4647 (24 hours, 365 days a year)
Website: www.nhsdirect.nhs.uk

Offers confidential health-care advice, information and referral service. A good first port of call for any health advice.

## NHS Smoking Helpline
Freephone: 0800 022 4332 (7am–11pm, 365 days a year)
Website: http://smokefree.nhs.uk
Pregnancy smoking helpline: 0800 169 9169
(12 noon–9pm, 365 days a year)

Have advice, help and encouragement on giving up smoking. Specialist advisers available to offer ongoing support to those who genuinely are trying to give up smoking. Can refer to local branches.

## Patients' Association
PO Box 935
Harrow, Middlesex HA1 3YJ
Helpline: 0845 608 4455
Tel: 020 8423 9111
Website: www.patients-association.com

Provides advice on patients' rights, leaflets and a directory of self-help groups.

## Quit (Smoking Quitlines)
63 St Mary's Axe
London EC3 8AA
Helpline: 0800 002200 (9am–9pm, 365 days a year)
Tel: 020 7469 0400
Website: www.quit.org.uk

Offers individual advice on giving up smoking in English and Asian languages. Talks to schools on smoking and pregnancy and can refer to local support groups. Runs training courses for professionals.

## Stroke Association
Stroke House
240 City Road
London EC1V 2PR
Tel: 020 7566 0300
Helpline: 0845 303 3100
Website: www.stroke.org.uk

Funds research and provides information, now specialising only in strokes. Local support groups.

## Vegetarian Society

Parkdale, Dunham Road
Altrincham, Cheshire WA14 4QG
Tel: 0161 925 2000 (Mon–Fri 8.30am–5pm)
Website: www.vegsoc.org

Provides a starter pack on the vegetarian way of life and information sheet about fats and cholesterol. Send an A5 SAE for a list of local groups and cookery books.

## Useful websites

### BBC

**www.bbc.co.uk/health**

A helpful website: easy to navigate and offers lots of useful advice and information. Also contains links to other related topics.

### NHS choices

**www.nhs.uk/conditions**

Government's patient information portal.

### Patient UK

**www.patient.co.uk**

Patient care website.

## The internet as a source of further information

After reading this book, you may feel that you would like further information on the subject. The internet is of course an excellent place to look and there are many websites with useful information about medical disorders, related charities and support groups.

It should always be remembered, however, that the internet is unregulated and anyone is free to set up a website and add information to it. Many websites offer impartial advice and information that has been compiled and checked by qualified medical professionals. Some, on the other hand, are run by commercial organisations with the purpose of promoting their own products. Others still are run by pressure groups, some of which will provide carefully assessed and accurate information whereas others may be suggesting medications or treatments that are not supported by the medical and scientific community.

Unless you know the address of the website you want to visit – for example, www.familydoctor.co.uk – you may find the following guidelines useful when searching the internet for information.

### Search engines and other searchable sites

Google (www.google.co.uk) is the most popular search engine used in the UK, followed by Yahoo! (http://uk.yahoo.com) and MSN (www.msn.co.uk). Also popular are the search engines provided by Internet Service Providers such as Tiscali and other sites such as the BBC site (www.bbc.co.uk).

In addition to the search engines that index the whole web, there are also medical sites with search facilities, which act almost like mini-search engines, but cover only medical topics or even a particular area of medicine. Again, it is wise to look at who is responsible for compiling the information offered to ensure that it is impartial and medically accurate. The NHS Direct site (www.nhsdirect.nhs.uk) is an example of a searchable medical site.

Links to many British medical charities can be found at the Association of Medical Research Charities' website (www.amrc.org.uk) and at Charity Choice (www.charitychoice.co.uk).

## Search phrases

Be specific when entering a search phrase. Searching for information on 'cancer' will return results for many different types of cancer as well as on cancer in general. You may even find sites offering astrological information. More useful results will be returned by using search phrases such as 'lung cancer' and 'treatments for lung cancer'. Both Google and Yahoo! offer an advanced search option that includes the ability to search for the exact phrase; enclosing the search phrase in quotes, that is, 'treatments for lung cancer', will have the same effect. Limiting a search to an exact phrase reduces the number of results returned but it is best to refine a search to an exact match only if you are not getting useful results with a normal search. Adding 'UK' to your search term will bring up mainly British sites, so a good phrase might be 'lung cancer' UK (don't include UK within the quotes).

Always remember the internet is international and unregulated. It holds a wealth of valuable information but individual sites may be biased, out of date or just plain wrong. Family Doctor Publications accepts no responsibility for the content of links published in this series.

# Index

# Your pages

We have included the following pages because they may help you manage your illness or condition and its treatment.

Before an appointment with a health professional, it can be useful to write down a short list of questions of things that you do not understand, so that you can make sure that you do not forget anything.

Some of the sections may not be relevant to your circumstances.

We are always pleased to receive constructive criticism or suggestions about how to improve the books. You can contact us at:

Email:   familydoctor@btinternet.com
Letter:  Family Doctor Publications
         PO Box 4664
         Poole
         BH15 1NN

*Thank you*

## Health-care contact details

Name:

Job title:

Place of work:


Tel:


Name:

Job title:

Place of work:


Tel:


Name:

Job title:

Place of work:


Tel:


Name:

Job title:

Place of work:


Tel:

## Significant past health events – illnesses/operations/investigations/treatments

| Event | Month | Year | Age (at time) |
|---|---|---|---|
| | | | |
| | | | |
| | | | |
| | | | |
| | | | |
| | | | |
| | | | |
| | | | |
| | | | |
| | | | |
| | | | |
| | | | |
| | | | |
| | | | |
| | | | |
| | | | |
| | | | |
| | | | |
| | | | |
| | | | |
| | | | |

## Appointments for health care

Name:

Place:

Date:

Time:

Tel:

Name:

Place:

Date:

Time:

Tel:

Name:

Place:

Date:

Time:

Tel:

Name:

Place:

Date:

Time:

Tel:

## Appointments for health care

Name:

Place:

Date:

Time:

Tel:

Name:

Place:

Date:

Time:

Tel:

Name:

Place:

Date:

Time:

Tel:

Name:

Place:

Date:

Time:

Tel:

## Current medication(s) prescribed by your doctor

Medicine name:

Purpose:

Frequency & dose:

Start date:

End date:

Medicine name:

Purpose:

Frequency & dose:

Start date:

End date:

Medicine name:

Purpose:

Frequency & dose:

Start date:

End date:

Medicine name:

Purpose:

Frequency & dose:

Start date:

End date:

## Other medicines/supplements you are taking, not prescribed by your doctor

Medicine/treatment:

Purpose:

Frequency & dose:

Start date:

End date:

Medicine/treatment:

Purpose:

Frequency & dose:

Start date:

End date:

Medicine/treatment:

Purpose:

Frequency & dose:

Start date:

End date:

Medicine/treatment:

Purpose:

Frequency & dose:

Start date:

End date:

## Questions to ask at appointments

(Note: do bear in mind that doctors work under great time
pressure, so long lists may not be helpful for either of you)

## Questions to ask at appointments

(Note: do bear in mind that doctors work under great time
pressure, so long lists may not be helpful for either of you)

# Notes

# Notes

# Notes